Population Ecotoxicology

Hierarchical Ecotoxicology Series

Editor

Michael C. Newman
College of William and Mary
Virginia Institute of Marine Science
Virginia
USA

Ecotoxicology is a rapidly expanding field of research within the international scientific community. Ecotoxicology is a hierarchical science, concerned simultaneously with several different levels of biological organization.

This series of five books takes each level of the biological hierarchy: Individuals, Population, Community, Ecosystem and Landscape, and the entire Biosphere and provides a primary source of information on the basic paradigms emerging at each level.

Each book will focus on one level at a time but also defines the connections between levels. Identification and discussion of ecotoxicological paradigms form the backbone for each book.

Forthcoming titles in the series

Ecotoxicology organismal
M. C. Newman

Community Ecotoxicology
W. Clements and M. C. Newman

Ecosystem and Landscape Ecotoxicology
M. C. Newman

Global Ecotoxicology
M. C. Newman

Population Ecotoxicology

MICHAEL C. NEWMAN
College of William and Mary, Virginia Institute of Marine Science, Virginia, USA

JOHN WILEY & SONS, LTD
Chichester • New York • Weinheim • Brisbane • Singapore • Toronto

Copyright © 2001 John Wiley & Sons, Ltd
Baffins Lane, Chichester,
West Sussex PO19 1UD, England

National   01243 779777
International (+44) 1243 779777
e-mail (for orders and customer service enquiries): cs-books@wiley.co.uk
Visit our Home Page on: http://www.wiley.co.uk
or http://www.wiley.com

Other Wiley Editorial Offices

John Wiley & Sons, Inc., 605 Third Avenue,
New York, NY 10158-0012, USA

Wiley-VCH Verlag GmbH, Pappelallee 3,
D-69469 Weinheim, Germany

John Wiley & Sons Australia, Ltd, 33 Park Road, Milton,
Queensland 4064, Australia

John Wiley & Sons (Asia) Pte Ltd, 2 Clementi Loop #02-01,
Jin Xing Distripark, Singapore 129809

John Wiley & Sons (Canada) Ltd, 22 Worcester Road,
Rexdale, Ontario M9W 1L1, Canada

British Library Cataloguing in Publication Data

A catalogue record for this book is available from the British Library

ISBN 0 471 98818 9

Typeset in 10/12pt Times from the author's disk by Laser Words, Madras, India
Printed and bound in Great Britain by Biddles Ltd, Guildford, Surrey
This book is printed on acid-free paper responsibly manufactured from sustainable forestry,
in which at least two trees are planted for each one used for paper production

Do that which will render thee worthy of happiness.
Critique of Pure Reason   (I. Kant 1781)

To my family,
Peg, Ben & Ian

Contents

Series Preface

This five-volume *Hierarchical Ecotoxicology Series* is intended to bridge a widening gap between general ecotoxicology textbooks and technical books focused on specific ecotoxicological topics. Important, narrowly focused books abound, and textbooks appear yearly but are necessarily broad treatments of the field of ecotoxicology. This series was conceived from the belief that a synthesis is needed that provides the student with an understanding beyond that afforded by a general textbook but, unlike that from more specialized books, remains focused on paradigms and fundamental methods.

This series has separate volumes for the ecotoxicology of individuals, populations, communities, ecosystems and landscapes, and the entire biosphere. Although these topics are treated separately, the intent is to integrate ecotoxicology as a science across these hierarchical levels.

Acknowledgements

The author is extremely grateful for the thoughtful chapter reviews contributed by the following people. Particularly helpful were the comprehensive reviews of all chapters by Margaret Mulvey and many chapters by Carl Strojan. Margaret Mulvey also produced Box 7.1 in Chapter 7.

Clements, William	Colorado State University
Crane, Mark	University of London — Royal Holloway
Dixon, Philip	Iowa State University
Mulvey, Margaret	College of William and Mary (VIMS)
Rench, Jerry	Research Triangle Institute
Strojan, Carl	University of Georgia (SREL)
Van Veld, Peter	College of William and Mary (VIMS)

1 The Hierarchical Science of Ecotoxicology

1.1 THE OVERARCHING CONTEXT OF HIERARCHICAL ECOTOXICOLOGY

1.1.1 GENERAL

Ecotoxicology is the science of contaminants in the biosphere and their effects on constituents of the biosphere, including humans (Newman 1998). The scope of ecotoxicology is so necessarily encompassing that an ecotoxicologist can study fate or effect of toxicants from the molecular to the biospheric scales. Therefore, it is necessary at the onset of this volume to give a context within which the field will be explored. The context and philosophical vantage for this volume — in fact for the entire series — are sketched out in this brief chapter. The themes discussed here will emerge throughout the series.

I have argued that there is intrinsically only one class of explanation. It traverses the scales of space, time, and complexity to unite the disparate facts of the disciplines by consilience, the perception of a seamless web of cause and effect. (Wilson 1998)

Wilson articulates a central theme of this series, that is, to provide detailed discussion of one level of biological organization at a time with a progressive interlinking of facts and paradigms among levels. Expressed in terms of conceptual systems theory, the series tries to foster the complementary processes of differentiation and integration. Differentiation is the ability to pull together a large number of diverse facts and concepts and to maintain discrimination among these facts and concepts (Karlins 1973). The series attempts to bring a student's capacity for differentiation beyond that provided in introductory textbooks. It also has the sister goal of integration, the interrelating of concepts and information from different levels into a coherent whole.

These two goals allow in-depth exploration of paradigms and important approaches at each level while emphasizing the complementary nature of information extracted from proximate levels. Too often, studies at different levels of biological organization are perceived as producing incompatible insights, or worse, as being competing systems of explanation (Maciorowski 1988). Conclusions from one level may be judged deficient based on criteria relevant to another level. Such self-imposed nearsightedness eventually assures that information produced in the context of one level cannot be translated to that of another without great difficulty and compromise. This conceptual myopia is a common, yet correctable, condition associated with complex topics.

> *As a question becomes more complicated and involved, and extends to a greater number of relations, disagreement of opinion will always be multiplied, not because we are irrational, but because we are finite beings, furnished with different kinds of knowledge, exerting different degrees of attention, one discovering consequences which escape another, none taking in the whole concatenation of causes and effects, and most comprehending but a very small part; each referring it to a different purpose. Where, then, is the wonder, that they, who see only a small part, should judge erroneously of the whole? Or that they, who see different and dissimilar parts, should judge differently from each other?* (Johnson 1753)

My fundamental premise in preparing this series is that optimal understanding is fostered by acquiring sound information, organizing it around explanations (paradigms) emerging at each level, and then, integrating information and paradigms into a consonant whole. This premise emerges partially from Nagel's (1961) argument that the goal of any science is to organize knowledge around explanatory principles. But more than this is required. For ecotoxicology, the knowledge to be organized emerges from the suborganismal to biospheric scales. I am convinced that, to be maximally useful, the organization of knowledge in ecotoxicology, as in any science, must be congruent among hierarchical levels of biological organization. While this may seem obvious, in practice it has been a difficult goal to obtain.

1.1.2 THE MODIFIED JANUS CONTEXT

How can organization and integration of knowledge be achieved? A straightforward approach will be applied to foster congruity in this hierarchical science. The first component of this approach was described by Koestler (1991). He defined the Janus effect or context for hierarchical, biological systems. (Janus was a Roman deity, who was often carved at doorways with two faces looking in opposite directions.) Like Janus, any level of the biological organization faces in two directions: it presents two faces simultaneously to the scientist. It is a whole composed of parts while also being a part of a larger whole. Such a unit or sub-assembly within a hierarchical system was called a holon by Koestler. I assume in this series that no hierarchical level (holon) has a favored status relative to causation or conceptual consonance.

The Janus context of Koestler (1991) is modified slightly here to include a simple, but awkwardly phrased, 'unfixed cause–effect–significance concatenation' scheme. Hereafter, this scheme is referred to simply as the unfixed concatenation scheme.

The unfixed concatenation scheme is common in many thoughtful treatments of hierarchical topics in the natural sciences. Simply stated, causal mechanisms explaining an observed effect at a particular level are sought at the level(s) immediately below it, while the significance of the effect is sought at the next higher level(s). For example, the observation of reproductive failure of individuals exposed to a pollutant — an observation at the organismal level — is explained by changes in endocrine function — a causal mechanism at the organ system level. The consequence or significance is sought at the population level, i.e. risk of local extinction of populations in polluted areas. This concatenation of cause–effect–significance is applied equally well to any level. Ideally, this unfixed concatenation permits a smooth conceptual transition from one level to another without experiencing what Kuhn (see Watkins 1970) calls an abrupt gestalt switch. In this case, the abrupt gestalt shift would be an incongruous transition from one set of level-specific paradigms to another. As Popper (1959) argued regarding self-contradictory groupings of paradigms, any system of explanations not affording a smooth transition from one level to another is uninformative in the short term and nonviable in the long term. In this series, I meld the unfixed concatenation theme with the Janus context to foster congruity of explanation.

> ...*there is a translation problem at the core of ecotoxicology: how to translate mechanisms at one level into effects of another. This problem is not unique to ecotoxicology, but arises in studies of any hierarchical system. In such systems, processes at one level take their mechanisms from the level below and find their consequences at the level above. The organismal physiology that is 'mechanistic detail' to a population biologist is the pattern that the physiologist wants to explain and a higher-level integration in the eyes of a biochemist. Recognizing this principle makes it clear that there are no truly 'fundamental' explanations, and makes it possible to move smoothly up and down the levels of a hierarchical system without falling into the traps of naive reductionism or pseudo-scientific holism.* (Caswell 1996)

A balancing note must follow this argument for the unfixed concatenation scheme. It should not blind ecotoxicologists to the occasionally appropriate cause–effect context that does not proceed upward monotonically through levels. For example, herbicide application to control forbs and shrub-grass on Colorado range land results in plant community composition shifts (Johnson and Hansen 1969). This change in habitat quality may produce territorial shifts and dominance-structure changes in an endemic rodent population, resulting in lowered population viability. The causal cascade can be viewed as initiated by change at the community level. Effects occurred at the population level with eventual consequences of diminished rodent population size. So, application of this useful context requires some temperance.

1.2 REDUCTIONISM VERSUS HOLISM DEBATE

1.2.1 REDUCTIONISM VERSUS HOLISM AS A FALSE DICHOTOMY

Merging aspects of mammalian toxicology and ecology in the initial framing of ecotoxicology resulted in a distracting debate about whether the reductionist or holist approach was best for dealing with ecotoxicological problems. In my opinion, few topics deserve to be ignored more than this one. However, it is a context that any informed reader will expect to be addressed, and therefore, an explanation for its absence in the series is needed. I argue that this debate is inconsistent with and dysfunctional within the context described above for deriving and organizing knowledge from hierarchical subjects. It also distracts students from much more important topics such as methods for improving the strength of inferences about ecotoxicological subjects. As we will see, the real difficulties are inference without information about emergent properties, inference without complete causal knowledge, and inference from aggregated information (i.e. the problem of ecological inference).

1.2.2 MICROEXPLANATION, HOLISM AND MACROEXPLANATION

Review of science philosophy provides a wider context for the reductionism–holism debate. What are usually identified as qualities of reductionism are those of microexplanation, where 'the properties and powers of individual things and of materials is due to their fine structure, that is due to the dispositions and interactions of their parts' (Harré 1972). Microexplanation, emerging from the corpuscularian concept of structure, holds that 'the global properties of individuals become functions of the properties of their parts' (Harré 1972). Within the context described above, this mode of exploring causation is very profitable. However, unique properties emerge at higher levels that are difficult or impossible to predict by microexplanation alone. Conceding the unpredictablity and importance of emergent properties in ecotoxicological systems, holism aims at describing consistent details and predictable behaviors of the whole without becoming completely entangled in a complex web of microexplanation. So, the holistic mode of generating information is also very profitable in the context just described. Finally, a third mode, macroexplanation, is also used to explain 'the nature and structure of the parts of an individual thing in terms of the characteristics of the whole thing' (Harré 1972). Inferences are made about the behavior of parts from the behavior of the whole, that is, from aggregate data. Macroexplanation is valuable also but has as significant problems (i.e. the problem of ecological inference discussed below) in its application as do holism and microexplanation.

Three, not two, investigative modes exist: microexplanation (reductionism), holism, and macroexplanation. In a hierarchical system, they can be envisioned as bottom → top, top → top, and top → bottom modes for understanding, respectively. In the modified Janus context, they are modes of inquiry applicable to the different 'faces' of any holon. It is inconceivable that exclusion of any one of the three would foster growth and continuity in ecotoxicology. Each has strengths when properly used and weaknesses when abused. Microexplanation assumes consequences of emergent properties are unimportant. Macroexplanation brings logical compromises by attempting to extract information on parts that is hidden within the measured properties of the whole. Such aggregated information makes inferences quite uncertain at times. Holistic descriptions of consistent relationships without knowledge of causal mechanisms can lead to ineffective extrapolation or prediction within and between levels.

To favor one mode of investigation is inconsistent within the modified Janus context. The cause at one level is the consistent association (e.g. chemical exposure–biological effect relationship) described at another. Identifying the significance at one level from a phenomenon observed at a lower one depends as much on the observation of a consistent association as on any mechanistic underpinnings. Holistic prediction based on consistency does not, and often cannot, require full mechanistic knowledge. Regardless, it is inherently limited without such mechanistic knowledge. In the modified Janus context, cause is sought at a lower level via reductionism after observation of a consistent association at a level. The initial observation of a consistent association was probably made in what many would describe as a holistic study. Some macroexplanation may have been applied based on paradigms from the next highest level. Macroexplanation is often applied to results from studies with a strong holistic context and is often the true root for contention between reductionists and holists.

1.2.3 A CLOSER LOOK AT MACROEXPLANATION

Macroexplanation requires more comment because it is not a topic much discussed by ecotoxicologists. It also contains a potential problem as large as the emergent properties problem so often thrust at reductionists by holists or the limited prediction problem thrust back at holists by reductionists. Although discussion of macroexplanation is often drowned out by the reductionism/holism banter, macroexplanation (top → bottom) is applied frequently in ecology and ecotoxicology. For example, a shift in population structure after pollution exposure may be used to infer how individual life history strategies may have changed, or used to formulate testable hypotheses about changes in reproduction or survival of individuals. Macroexplanation is common when natural selection theory is invoked to suggest how individuals optimize their fitness under stressful conditions. This 'process of using aggregate (i.e. "ecological") data to infer individual-level relationships of interest when individual-level data are not available' (King 1997) is called ecological inference in sociology (King 1997) and epidemiology (Last 1983). (Notice that 'ecological' denotes only that the data are aggregate in nature. Etymology aside, it has nothing to do with the subject of ecology.)

Ecological inference is used by social scientists and epidemiologists with extreme care and difficulty. King (1997) gives the example of difficulties in inferring how individual women voted on a particular equal rights bill based solely on aggregated knowledge of voting outcome and the gender composition for voting precincts. Without direct knowledge of how individual women voted, correlations are generated between proportion of all voters who were women versus the proportion of all voters supporting the bill in a precinct. Several explanations are possible for a positive correlation between proportion of voters who were women and the proportion who voted for the bill in a precinct. Perhaps individual women tended to vote for the bill. Alternatively, and not necessarily exclusive of this first explanation, the voting pattern of individual men might have changed to produce a correlation and female voting behavior remained relatively constant among precincts. Competing explanations cannot be easily culled away because essential information was lost to aggregation, i.e., the process of anonymous voting. More relevant examples emerge in epidemiology. Radon levels measured in counties and lung cancer deaths tallied in these counties may be used to imply the chances of an individual dying of lung cancer at a certain radon exposure concentration (King 1997). Similarly, correlations between water quality in regions of the USA and heart disease may be used to estimate risk of heart disease for an individual living in a region with water hardness of a certain level (Last 1983). With the application of ecological inference, there is a risk that a researcher's predilection will be used inappropriately to identify the 'best' explanation when alternate explanations are possible. This is the ecological fallacy or problem of ecological inference.

The ecological inference problem emerges in many ecotoxicological studies of aggregated data. For example, the DEBtox program (Kooijman and Bedaux 1996) uses theoretical equations to estimate toxicant elimination rate constants based on the mortality of animals in toxicity tests. Elimination kinetics are not measured and must be mathematically implied from aggregate data, i.e. lethal and sublethal effects to individuals held at various toxicant concentrations. In surprising contrast to the careful attention paid to this problem in the social sciences, it appears without much debate or comment in ecotoxicology. When the problem of ecological inference is raised, it is usually misidentified as a basic flaw of holism. Perhaps our preoccupation with the reductionism/holism debate contributes to this neglect. As a scientist inclined more toward reductionism than holism, the logical difficulty of using aggregated information derived in a holistic study to suggest a mechanism at the next lowest level (i.e. the problem of ecological inference) makes me hesitate before designing a holistic or descriptive study. (Note that the data would only be considered aggregate if they were used to suggest behavior of parts at one level down from that being measured.) The problem of ecological inference can appear while attempting to extract more information from holistic studies generating 'aggregate' data. This is the reductionist's counter-argument to the inability to predict emergent properties with a predominantly reductionist approach. The optimal solution for ecotoxicology is to use all approaches thoughtfully and to avoid their over extension, i.e. acknowledge the problem of ecological inference, limits of prediction from holistic analysis, and the possibility of emergent properties.

1.3 REQUIREMENTS IN THE SCIENCE OF ECOTOXICOLOGY

1.3.1 GENERAL

Let's assume that the modified Janus context is the correct one for planning ecotoxicological research programs and for organizing knowledge around ecotoxicological paradigms. The reductionism/holism debate becomes immediately irrelevant because the modified Janus context implies that all levels are equally valid foci for exploring the cause–effect–significance concatenation. For any level, one needs to understand its parts and also how that level functions as part of a larger whole. This can only be done by simultaneous and thoughtful application of microexplanation, holism and macroexplanation. These observational modes are equally useful to all levels of organization because no level has a favored status and the cause–effect–significance structure can be shifted freely to any level. This conclusion is contrary to current dogma that reductionism is more applicable at lower levels and holism is more useful at higher levels. Hopefully, the distraction of such confused conclusions from the reductionism/holism debate is now gone and we can move on to more useful topics.

What is most needed in ecotoxicology is the accumulation of high-quality knowledge and the structuring of that knowledge around rigorously tested explanatory principles. Further, the present chimerical state of knowledge must be slowly transformed to foster consilience of explanatory principles (paradigms) among levels organization. Without these changes, ecotoxicologists remain scientific jerry-builders.

How can one assess the relative value of research programs in accomplishing these goals if it doesn't matter what level of biological organization is being addressed, or whether a reductionist or holist stance is taken? I believe that assessment of relative value for most hierarchical sciences is surprisingly straightforward if based on two qualities: the strength of associated inferences and consilience among paradigms. Consilience has already been discussed so inferential strength is the only component needing further explanation.

1.3.2 STRONG INFERENCE

The concept of strong inference is described in a remarkable article by Platt (1964). At the heart of strong inference is the Baconian scientific method. A working hypothesis and alternate hypothesis are formulated, and a discriminating experiment is performed. The result is used to produce additional hypotheses and the process repeated until only one hypothesis remains as a viable explanation for the observations. This process guides a researcher through a dichotomous logic tree to a final explanation for the phenomenon under study. The strong inference process extends this method. The concept of multiple working hypotheses (Chamberlin 1897) is added because the Baconian method tends to favor a central hypothesis in the formulation of tests and to bias the allocation of effort toward this favored hypothesis during the falsification process. An unintentional bias emerges with the tendency for investigators to feel ownership for a particular hypothesis or explanation. Chamberlin's solution was to advocate a multiple working hypothesis framework. All reasonable hypotheses are formulated and experimental effort spent equitably among these hypotheses. This process diminishes the tendency to become enamored with a particular explanation and shifts the emphasis to the process of discriminating among the candidate hypotheses. The researcher owns the process, not a favored hypothesis or explanation. This process also reduces the tendency to stop testing when 'the cause' is discovered, where in fact, there might be multiple causes for a phenomenon. The final and crucial aspect of strong inference is that the process must be taught and practiced consistently in the field. Using an analogy, Platt (1964) explains the benefits of this approach relative to the rate at which a scientific field can advance.

> *The difference between the average scientist's informal methods and the methods of the strong-inference users is somewhat like the difference between a gasoline engine that fires occasionally and one that fires in steady sequence. If our motorboat engines were as erratic as our deliberate intellectual efforts, most of us would not get home for supper.*

I can suggest only one improvement to Platt's strong inference approach. Although all effort should be made to perform tests that result in clear dichotomous outcomes, e.g. reject or do not reject the hypothesis, the discrimination afforded by many formal experiments and less structured, observational studies is often less clear. The dichotomous falsification process described for the strong inference approach can be enhanced by including abductive inference — inference to the best explanation (Josephson and Josephson 1996). Modern statistical methods, especially Bayesian methods, allow the conclusion that a hypothesis is falsified when it becomes sufficiently improbable. A 'reject/accept' conclusion from hypothesis tests is no longer essential for rigorously evaluating an explanation. This final modification produces an extremely powerful approach for making strong inferences in ecotoxicology and, consequently, for accelerating advancement in the field. Strong inference is equally valuable for all levels of the ecotoxicological hierarchy and investigative modes.

1.4 SUMMARY

My intent in producing this *Hierarchical Ecotoxicology Series* is to bridge a gap opening between general textbooks and highly specialized books. My conceptual tack is to provide more details about key paradigms and approaches, and to explore the consilience possible among levels of organization. The stagnant reductionism/holism context is rejected in favor of a modified Janus context. Based on this context, the cause–effect–significance sequence can slide freely up and down the scales of this hierarchical science. The three modes of investigation (microexplanation, macroexplanation and holism) are relevant at all levels of biological organization. Strong inference augmented by modern techniques of abductive inference is advocated as the best investigative mode in this new science. I believe that our collective commitment to strong inference and conceptual consilience will determine whether or not ecotoxicology quickly realizes its potential for becoming one of the most important sciences of the new millennium.

1.4.1 SUMMARY OF FOUNDATION CONCEPTS AND PARADIGMS

- Ecotoxicology is the science of contaminants in the biosphere and their effects on constituents of the biosphere, including humans.
- Ecotoxicology is a hierarchical science.
- No level in the ecotoxicological hierarchy is better than another relative to identifying causation or attributing relevance.
- Essential to the growth of ecotoxicology are (a) application of strong inference to efficiently organize knowledge around rigorously tested paradigms (explanatory principals), and (b) consilience of concepts and paradigms among all hierarchical levels.
- The modified Janus context allows optimal inference and organization of knowledge around paradigms at all levels of biological organization.
- Wider application of the methods of strong inference, perhaps adding modern methods of abductive inference, would greatly accelerate progress in ecotoxicology.
- Current ecotoxicological knowledge is often incongruous among levels of organization.
- The holism–reductionism debate is invalid and a distraction.
- Three modes of acquiring knowledge and enhancing belief are useful: microexplanation (reductionism), macroexplanation (inference about parts from the behavior of the whole), and holism (inference from observation of a consistent pattern or behavior without the requirement of a lower level, causal explanation).
- Inference based on holism may lead to prediction error as causal mechanisms are not necessarily known.
- Inference based on microexplanation (reductionism) may lead to prediction error as properties difficult or impossible to predict can emerge at higher levels of organization.
- Inference based on macroexplanation may lead to prediction error due to the problem of ecological inference.

REFERENCES

Caswell H (1996). Demography meets ecotoxicology: Untangling the population level effects of toxic substances. In *Ecotoxicology. A Hierarchical Treatment*, ed. by MC Newman and CH Jagoe, pp. 255–292. CRC/Lewis Publishers, Boca Raton, FL.

Chamberlin TC (1897). The method of multiple working hypotheses. *J Geol* **5**: 837–848.

Harré R (1972). *The Philosophies of Science. An Introductory Survey*. Oxford University Press, Oxford.

Johnson S (1753). The Adventurer. In 1968. *Samuel Johnson. Selected Writings*, ed. by P Cruttwell, pp. 186–204. Penguin Books, London (1968).

Johnson DR and Hansen RM (1969). Effects of range treatment with 2,4-D on rodent populations. *J Wildl Manage* **33**:125–132.

Josephson JR and SG Josephson (1996). *Abductive Inference. Computation, Philosophy, Technology*. Cambridge University Press, Cambridge.

Karlins M (1973). Conceptual complexity and remote-associative proficiency as creativity variables in a complex problem-solving task. In *Creativity. Theory and Research*, ed. by M Bloomberg pp. 200–228. College & University Press, New Haven, CT.

King G (1997). *A Solution to the Ecological Inference Problem*. Princeton University Press, Princeton, NJ.

Koestler A (1991). Holons and hierarchy theory. In *From Gaia to Selfish Gene. Selected Writings in the Life Sciences*, ed. by C Barlow pp. 88–100. The MIT Press, Cambridge, MA.

Kooijman SALM and Bedaux JJM (1996). *The Analysis of Aquatic Toxicity Data*. VU University Press, Amsterdam.

Last JM (1983). *A Dictionary of Epidemiology*. Oxford University Press, New York.

Maciorowski AF (1988). Populations and communities: linking toxicology and ecology in a new synthesis. *Environ Toxicol Chem* **7**:677–678.

Nagel E (1961). *The Structure of Science. Problems in the Logic of Scientific Explanation*. Harcourt, Brace and World, New York.

Newman MC (1998). *Fundamentals of Ecotoxicology*. Ann Arbor Press, Chelsea, MI.

Platt JR (1964). Strong inference. *Science* **146**: 347–353.

Popper KR (1959). *The Logic of Scientific Discovery*. T.J. Press (Padstow) Ltd, London.

Watkins J (1970). Against 'Normal Science'. In *Criticism and the Growth of Knowledge* ed. by I Lakatos and A Musgrave pp. 25–37. Cambridge University Press, Cambridge.

Wilson EO (1998). *Consilience*. Alfred A. Knopf, New York.

2 The Population Ecotoxicology Context

The emergence of ecological toxicology as a coherent discipline is perhaps unique in that it combines aspects of toxicology and ecology, both of which are in and of themselves synthetic sciences...Chemicals may affect every level of biological organization (molecules, cells, tissues, organs, organ systems, organisms, populations, communities) contained in ecosystems. Any one of these levels is a potential unit of study for the field, as are the interdependent structures and relationships within and between levels. (Maciorowski 1988)

2.1 POPULATION ECOTOXICOLOGY DEFINED

2.1.1 WHAT IS ECOTOXICOLOGY?

Ecotoxicology, a science combining ecology and toxicology, may encompass slightly different things depending on a particular practitioner's training. Often, those trained in classic toxicology emphasize the lower levels of biological organization. They explore biochemical and cellular mechanisms; perhaps, using this knowledge to develop valuable biomarkers of toxicant exposure or effect. Ecotoxicologists trained in ecology during the last few decades emphasize the ecosystem context and study the behavior of ecosystem components under the influence of toxicants. There are also some practitioners with training in biogeochemistry who focus on toxicant fate and transport in the environment. They may or may not confine themselves to the ecosystem context. Although there are disadvantages to this plurality within our discipline and some confusion emerges from the inappropriate application of methods borrowed from other fields, the overall result is a robust selection of vantages from which to discover facts and organize knowledge.

The variety of definitions of ecotoxicology that appear in the literature reflect this diversity. A comparison of definitions reveals that all possess the same core concept with slight differences in emphasis (see Table 1.2 in Newman (1998)). As discussed in Chapter 1, ecotoxicology is defined here as the science of contaminants in the biosphere and their effects on constituents of the biosphere, including humans.

The key terms in this definition requiring some brief comment are science, biosphere, constituents of the biosphere, and humans. We will emphasize in this series the scientific, not regulatory, aspects of ecotoxicology. Therefore, ecotoxicology is defined as a science. Until recently, the training of ecologists emphasized the ecosystem yet this context is now too small to hold all relevant topics. The biosphere is emphasized in the definition so that topics such as global movement of volatile organic compounds, acid precipitation, and landscape degradation can be included. Any narrower focus impedes understanding. Components of the biosphere will be considered in the hierarchical context described in Chapter 1. Finally, mechanisms and effects to humans are included in discussions when they are relevant. Artificially excising one species from consideration in organizing ecotoxicological knowledge seems excessive deference to recent tradition in this young field, especially if that species is the source of contaminants and the subject of much toxicological study.

2.1.2 WHAT IS A POPULATION?

Context and intent influence one's definition of a species population. An ecologist might visualize a population as a collection of individuals of the same species that occupy the same space at the same time. Suggested in this definition is a distinct boundary defining some space where, in fact, no such boundary may exist. So the spatial context for a population can be strict or operational depending on how clear spatial boundaries are. The temporal context for a population may be blurry too. Groups of individuals of the same species may come together and disperse through time, making it difficult to distinguish populations.

A more realistic image of many populations emerges if one considers the dynamics of a group of contemporaneous individuals of the same species occupying a habitat with patches differing markedly in their capacity to foster survival, growth, and reproduction. Differences among patches produce differences in fitnesses of individuals. Good habitat in the mosaic is a source of individuals because excess production of young is possible, while less favorable habitat is a sink for these excess individuals. A population living within such a habitat mosaic is called a metapopulation. The dynamics of metapopulations in source–sink habitats have unique features that should be understood by ecotoxicologists. For example, a sink habitat created by contamination may still possess high numbers of individuals, a condition inexplicable based on conventional ecotoxicity test results but easily explained in a metapopulation context. Also, the loss of a small area of land to contamination can have dire consequences if the lost land was a source habitat sustaining the metapopulation components in adjacent, clean habitats. Such keystone habitats are crucial for maintaining the population in adjacent areas and some species are particularly sensitive to loss of keystone habitat (O'Connor 1996).

The above concept of a population requires one more quality to be complete. A population is a collection of individuals of the same species occupying the same space at the same time and within which individuals may exchange genetic information (Odum 1971). Gene flow should be included in the identification of population boundaries. Population boundaries can be clear (e.g. a pupfish species in an isolated desert spring) or necessarily operational (e.g. mosquitofish in a stream branch). Spatial clines in gene flow become common because individuals in populations are more likely to mate with nearby neighbors than with more distant neighbors. Temporal changes in population boundaries must be considered. As an extreme example, if females store sperm and a toxicant kills all males after the breeding season, the dead males are still part of the effective population contributing genes to the next generation.

Mitton (1997) provides an additional context for populations that is relevant to population ecotoxicology. A species population can be studied in the context of all existing individuals throughout the species' range. The influence of some contaminant, alone or in combination with factors such as habitat loss or fragmentation, might be suspected as the cause of a species' decline or imminent extinction over its entire range. Such a broad biogeographical perspective is at the heart of one explanation for the current rapid decline in many amphibian populations throughout the biosphere. Sarokin and Schulkin (1992) describe several other instances of large-scale population changes and suggest potential linkage to widespread contaminants. In these instances, the population of concern is the entire collection of individuals comprising the species, not a local population. Assuming that toxicant-linked extinctions are undesirable, there is obvious value to studying the influence of contaminants on the biogeographic distribution and character of populations.

2.1.3 DEFINITION OF POPULATION ECOTOXICOLOGY

Population ecotoxicology is the science of contaminants in the biosphere and their effects on populations. In this book, a population is defined as a collection of contemporaneous individuals of the same species occupying the same space and within which genetic information may be exchanged. Population ecotoxicology considers contaminant effects in the context of epidemiology, basic demography, metapopulation biology, life history theory, and population genetics. Accordingly, the chapters of this volume are organized into these topics.

2.2 THE NEED FOR POPULATION ECOTOXICOLOGY

2.2.1 GENERAL

Why commit an entire book to population ecotoxicology? Is there sufficient merit to develop a population context to this science and to imposing this context on our present methods of environmental stewardship? The answers to these questions are easily formulated based on the scientific and practical advantages of doing so.

Although not often envisioned as such, landmark studies in population biology (e.g. population dynamics of agricultural pests) and evolutionary genetics (e.g. industrial melanism) involved pollutants. These ecotoxicological topics are currently associated with other disciplines such as population ecology and genetics because ecotoxicology is only now emerging as a distinct science and researchers who did those studies were affiliated with more established disciplines. Toxicants served as useful probes for teasing meaning from wild populations. Just as individuals with metabolic dysfunctions are studied by biochemists to better understand the metabolic processes taking place within healthy individuals, populations exposed to toxicants help us to understand the behavior of healthy populations. Often, they provide an accelerated look at processes such as natural selection, adaptation, and evolution that usually occur over time periods too long to study directly.

Equally clear are the practical advantages of better understanding toxicant effects to populations. Early problems involving pollutants centered on impacted populations. Widespread applications of DDT (2,2-bis-[p-chlorophenyl]-1,1,1-trichloroethane) and DDD (1,1-dichloro-2,2-bis-[p-chorophenyl] ethane) had unacceptable consequences to populations of predatory birds. Within 15 years of Paul Müeller receiving the 1948 Nobel Prize in medicine for discovering the insecticidal qualities of DDT, convincing evidence was mounting worldwide about declines in populations of raptors and fish-eating birds induced by DDT and its degradation product, DDE (1,1-dichloro-2,2-bis-[p-chlorophenyl]-ethene) (Dolphin 1959; Carson 1962; Hickey and Anderson 1968; Ratcliffe 1967, 1970; Woodwell, Wurster and Isaacson 1967).

Our current environmental concerns remain focused on population viability. Important examples include the presently unexplained drop in amphibian populations throughout the world (Wake 1991), the decline in British bird populations putatively due to widespread pesticide use (Beaumont 1997), and the population consequences of estrogenic chemicals (Fry and Toone 1981; Luoma 1992; McLachlan 1993). These concerns are predictable manifestations of the general displacement of species populations as the human population expanded to 'currently use 20 to 40% of the solar energy that is captured in organic materials by land plants' (Brown and Maurer 1989). This level of consumption by humans and the manner in which it is practiced could not but impact other species populations.

More and more authors are expressing the importance of population-level information in making environmental decisions, e.g. '...the effects of concern to ecologists performing assessments are those of long-term exposures on the persistence, abundance, and/or production of populations' (Barnthouse et al. 1987) and 'Environmental policy decision makers have shifted emphasis from physiological, individual-level to population-level impacts of human activities' (Emlen 1989). The phrasing of many federal laws and regulations likewise reflects this central concern for populations.

During the past two decades, toxicological endpoints (e.g., acute and chronic toxicity) for individual organisms have been the benchmarks for regulations and assessments of adverse ecological effects...The question most often asked regarding these data and their use in ecological risk assessment is, 'What is the significance of these ecotoxicity data to the integrity of the population?' More important, can we project or predict what happens to a pollutant-stressed population when biotic and abiotic factors are operating simultaneously in the environment?

Protecting populations is an explicitly stated goal of several Congressional and [Environmental Protection] *Agency mandates and regulations. Thus it is important that ecological risk assessment guidelines focus upon the protection and management at the population, community, and ecosystem levels...* (EPA 1991)

The practical value of using population-level tools in ecotoxicology is also clear in risk assessment. Both human and ecological risk assessments draw methods from epidemiology, the science of disease in populations. Epidemiological methods were applied in the Minamata Bay area to root out the cause for a mysterious disease in the local population. Since this early outbreak of pollutant-induced disease in a human population, epidemiology has become crucial in fostering human health in an environment containing complex mixtures of contaminants. Although used much less than warranted, epidemiological methods could be equally helpful in studying nonhuman populations.

2.2.2 SCIENTIFIC MERIT

So many examples come immediately to mind in considering the scientific merit of population ecotoxicology that the issue becomes selecting the best, not finding a convincing one. Natural selection in wild populations seems the most general illustration. Industrial melanism, a topic described in nearly all biology textbooks, is a population-level consequence of air pollution (Box 2.1). 'Industrial melanism in the peppered moth *(Biston betularia)* is the classic example of observable evolution by natural selection' (Grant *et al.* 1998). Further, the evolution of metal tolerance in plant species growing on mining waste is a clear example of natural selection in plants (Antonovics, Bradshaw and Turner 1971). Numerous additional examples of toxicant-driven microevolution include rodenticide resistance (Webb and Horsfall 1967; Bishop and Hartley 1976; Bishop, Hartley and Partridge 1977), insecticide resistance in target species (Comins 1977; Whitton Dearn and McKenzie 1980; McKenzie and Batterham 1994) and nontarget species resistance to toxicants (Boyd and Ferguson 1964; Klerks and Weis 1987; Weis and Weis 1989). It appears that, with the important exception of sickle cell anemia in human populations, the clearest and best-known examples of microevolution are those associated with anthropogenic toxicants.

Box 2.1   Industrial melanism — there and back again (almost)

Industrial melanism is universally acknowledged as one of the harbingers of our initial failure to create an industrial society compatible with ecological systems. Less well known, and perhaps as important, it is also one of the clearest indicators of a widespread improvement in air quality (Figure 2.1). Recent shifts in the occurrence of the color morphs of the peppered moth, *Biston betularia*, (Figure 2.2), suggest that the money and effort put into controlling air pollutants in several industrialized countries are having positive effects on air quality.

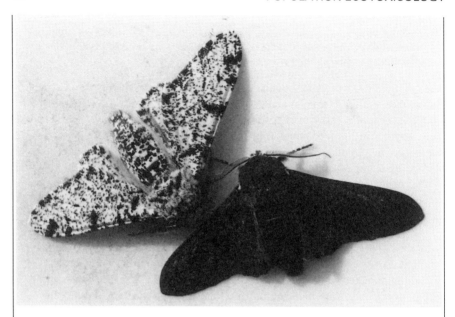

Fig. 2.1. Normal and melanistic color morphs of the peppered moth, *Biston betularia*. (Photograph courtesy of Bruce S. Grant, College of William & Mary)

Prior to around 1848, melanistic (dark-colored) morphs of the peppered moth were extremely rare. The conventional, and still sound, explanation for this observation is that (1) while quiescent during the day, this moth depends on its coloration to blend into its background, (2) this crypsis is focused on avoiding notice by visual predators, especially birds, (3) light coloration favors the moth if it rests on natural vegetation including light-colored lichens, (4) dark morphs appear due to mutation, but rarely, (5) dark morphs are less cryptic than light morphs relative to evading visual predators, (6) rare dark morphs are quickly taken by visual predators and, consequently, (7) light morphs predominate as rare dark morphs quickly disappear from natural populations (Kettlewell 1973).

British industrialization of the nineteenth century changed this situation by producing air pollutants that darkened surfaces and lowered the surface coverage by light-colored lichens. Crypsis began to favor the dark or *carbonaria* morph, and birds took more and more light morphs. The shift from a preponderance of light to dark moths was quite rapid because of large fitness differences among color morphs relative to avoiding notice of predators and the genetic dominance of the *carbonaria* allele over those for light morphs. (The light phenotypes are controlled by four recessive genes producing various pale to intermediate phenotypes (Lees and Creed 1977; Berry 1990).) Whereas one dark moth was observed around Manchester in 1848, moths of that area were composed almost entirely of dark morphs by 1895 (Clarke, Mani and Wynne 1985).

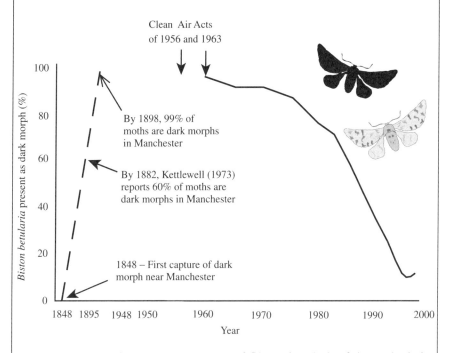

Fig. 2.2. Rise and fall in the proportion of *Biston betularia* of the melanistic morph caught near Liverpool, UK. Information for the decline in the dark morph come from Clarke and Grant (Clarke *et al.* 1994; Grant and Clarke 1999) who monitored a moth population outside of Liverpool from 1959 to the present

A subsequent series of events resulted in a second shift in the balance between light and dark morphs. Unacceptable consequences of poor air quality (including human and livestock illness and death) in the United Kingdom resulted in the passage and implementation of the 1956 and 1963 British Clean Air Acts (Grant, Owen and Clarke 1995). Air quality improved and dark morphs began to rapidly decline in numbers. In a comprehensive documentation of this change, Clarke and Grant (Clarke *et al.* 1994; Grant and Clarke 1999) report the clear decline in dark morphs from 1959 to present at Caldy Common, a location about 18 kilometers outside of Liverpool (Figure 2.2). The frequency of the dark morph dropped quickly until 1996 but, thereafter, fluctuated in the range of 7.1 to 11.5% (Grant and Clarke 1999). A similar leveling off at a low frequency occurred at a Nottingham location (Grant and Clarke 1999). Thus, although the population appears to be recovering, the moths have not returned to their pre-industrial state where the frequency of the *carbonaria* morph was extremely low. Perhaps there is a final part to this story yet to be written based on this new state with a low proportion of the once-rare, dark morph persisting in moth populations.

Biston betularia is an extremely widespread species and similar declines in pollution-related melanism have been documented in other countries (e.g. the United States (West 1977; Grant *et al* 1995, 1998) and The Netherlands (Brakefield 1990)) after enactment of air-quality legislation. When air quality improved, the frequency of the *carbonaria* morph declined. Peppered moth populations in Japan provide the exception that proves the rule. In Japan, unlike European industrial areas, the distribution of moths and industry were distinct. Thus, the conditions leading to the industrial melanism in other countries did not occur there (Asami and Grant 1994). Japanese studies serve as persuasive, negative controls for assessment of the relationship between pollution and melanism in *B. betularia* populations.

The story of industrial melanism continues. A significant proportion of all *B. betularia* in relevant British and US populations are still the *carbonaria* morph. Perhaps the dark morph will again become rare with further improvements in air quality. Perhaps not. Recent studies (Grant and Howlett 1988) indicate that Kettlewell's explanation based primarily on differential predation on adults by birds (Kettlewell 1955, 1973) may not be the complete story. The pre-adult stage has differences in viability (i.e. survival) fitness among color morphs (Mani 1990). Genetic shifts may be at least partially due to processes affecting pre-adults, i.e. nonvisual selection (Mani 1990). Further, multivariate statistical studies suggest that the best correlation between *B. betularia carbonaria* frequency in moth populations and air quality is with sulfur dioxide (Mani 1990; Grant *et al*. 1998). Although there is considerable opportunity for the problem of ecological inference to emerge here (see Chapter 1), it is possible that other mechanisms of selection associated with sulfur dioxide's effect on plants and animals might be important (e.g. acid precipitation-related direct changes to larval fitness or indirect effects by influencing vegetation quality). This classic example of population response to pollutants will likely yield more valuable insights as studies continue.

2.2.3 PRACTICAL MERIT

Extrapolations from laboratory bioassays to response in natural systems at the population level are effective if the environmental realism of the bioassay is sufficiently high. When laboratory systems are poor simulations of natural systems, gross extrapolation errors may result. The problem of extrapolating among levels of biological organization has not been given the serious attention its deserves. (Cairns and Pratt 1989)

Examples of the practical application of population ecotoxicology are also easily enumerated. They range from demographic analyses of toxicity test data (Karås, Neuman and Sandström 1991; Pesch, Munns and Gutjahr-Gobell 1991; Postma, van Kleunen and Admiraal 1995; Mulvey *et al.* 1995; Green and Chandler 1996; Caswell 1996) to surveys of field population qualities (Ginzburg *et al.* 1984; Sierszen and Frost 1993) to epidemiological analysis of populations in polluted areas (Hickey and Anderson 1968; Spitzer *et al.* 1978; Osowski *et al.* 1995) to using enhanced tolerance as an indicator of pollutant effect (Beardmore 1980; Klerks and Weis 1987; Mulvey and Diamond 1991; Guttman 1994). What follows is an illustration of the consequences of *not* considering population-level metrics of effect in practical ecotoxicology. The example illustrates the logical flaws incurred during predictions of effects to populations based on conventional toxicity test results.

Current ecotoxicity test methods have their roots in mammalian toxicology. Methods developed to infer the mammalian toxicity of various chemicals focused initially on lethal thresholds (Gaddum 1953). A dose or concentration was estimated below which no mortality would be expected. Because the statistical error associated with such a metric was quite high, effort shifted toward identification of a dose or concentration killing a certain percentage of exposed individuals, e.g. the LD50 or LC50 (Trevan 1927). A metric of toxicity was generated with a relatively narrow confidence interval. This proved suitable for measuring relative toxicity among chemicals or for the same chemical under different exposure situations. Ecotoxicologists adopted this approach *circa* mid-1940s to mid-1950s (Cairns and Pratt 1989) as a measure of toxicant effect (Maciorowski 1988; Cairns and Pratt 1989). To improve the metric, details such as different exposure durations (i.e. acute LC50 and chronic LC50), pathways (e.g. oral LC50 and dissolved LC50), and life stages (i.e. larval LC50, juvenile LC50, and adult LC50) were added. By the 1960s, these were the metrics of effect on organisms exposed to environmental toxicants that were 'generally accepted as a conservative estimate of the potential effects of test materials in the field' (Parrish 1985). These tests were extended further to predict field consequences of toxicant release by focusing testing on the most sensitive stage of a species' life cycle, e.g. early life stage tests.

Can tests that use such responses of individuals provide sufficiently accurate predictions of consequences to populations? Does the application of a metric that is not focused on population qualities compromise our ability to predict consequences to field populations? Four problems of using these metrics to predict population consequences come immediately to mind.

First, toxicity test interpretation is often based on the most sensitive life stage paradigm: if the most sensitive stage of an individual is protected, the species population will be protected. However, the most sensitive stage of the life history might not be the most crucial for maintaining a viable population (Petersen and Petersen 1988; Hopkin 1993). Newman (1998) uses the term 'weakest link incongruity' for this false assumption that the most sensitive stage of an individual's life history is the most crucial to population viability. For many species, there is an overproduction of individuals at the sensitive early life stage. Loss of sexually mature individuals might be more damaging to population persistence than a much higher loss of neonates. The loss of 10% of oyster larvae from a spawn may be trivial to the maintenance of a viable oyster population because oyster populations can accommodate wide fluctuations in annual spawning success. At the other extreme, sparrow hawk (kestrel) populations remain viable despite a loss of 60% of breeding females each year (Hopkin 1993). As a more ecotoxicological example, the most sensitive stage of the nematode, *Plectus acuminatus*, was not the most crucial stage in determining population effects of cadmium exposure (Kammenga *et al.* 1996). Inattention to population parameters creates a practical problem in prediction from ecotoxicity test results.

Second, metrics such as the 96 h LC50 cannot be fit into ordinary demographic analyses without introducing gross imprecision. Life tables require mortality information over the life time of a typical individual but LCx (or NOEC) metrics derived from one or a few observation times during the test are inadequate for filling in a life table. This problem would be greatly reduced if survival time models were produced from toxicity tests of the appropriate duration instead of a LC50 calculated for some set time (Dixon and Newman 1991; Newman and Aplin 1992; Newman and Dixon 1996; Newman and McCloskey 1996). Appropriate methods exist but are used rarely because of our preoccupation with metrics of toxicity to individuals without true concern for translation to the next hierarchical level, the population. This preoccupation with a traditional, statistically reliable metric of toxicity to individuals confounds appropriate analysis of mortality data and accurate prediction of population-level effects.

Third, although of less import when applying LC50-like metrics to determine toxicity in mammalian studies, post-exposure mortality of individuals exposed to a toxicant can make predictions of population-level effects grossly inaccurate based on a LC50-like metric. Considerable mortality can occur for many toxicants after exposure ends. As an example, 12% of mosquitofish (*Gambusia holbrooki*) exposed to 13 g/L of NaCl died by 144 h of exposure but another 44% died in the weeks immediately following termination of exposure (Newman and McCloskey 2000). Roughly 27% of mosquitofish exposed for 24 h to 500 μg/L pentachlorophenol died with an additional 15% dying in the week after exposure cessation (Newman and McCloskey 2000). This post-exposure mortality is irrelevant in the use of the LC50-like metrics in mammalian toxicology to measure relative toxicity but is extremely important in ecotoxicology where the population consequences of exposure are to be predicted. Post-exposure mortality in a population cannot continue to be treated as irrelevant in ecotoxicology.

Finally, as described in Box 2.2, the preoccupation with toxicity metrics borrowed from mammalian toxicology has distracted ecotoxicologists from important ambiguities about the underpinnings of the models used to predict effect. Ecotoxicology textbooks (e.g., Connell and Miller 1984; Landis and Yu 1995) and technical books (e.g. Finney 1947; Suter 1993; Forbes and Forbes 1994) explain the most widely used model (log normal or probit model) for concentration (or dose)-effect data with the individual tolerance or individual effective dose concept. The development of this model assumes that each individual has an innate dose at or above which it will die. The distribution of individual effective doses in a population is thought to be a log normal one. However, another explanation for observed log normal distributions is that the same stochastic processes are occurring in all individuals. The probability of dying is the same for all individuals and is best described by a log normal distribution. These two alternative hypotheses remain poorly tested but, in the context of population consequences of toxicant exposure, result in very different predictions (Box 2.2).

Practical problems emerge due to our preoccupation with measuring effects in a way more appropriate for predicting fate of exposed individuals than of exposed populations. In my opinion, current tests to predict population-level consequences are no less peculiar than one described in the poem *Science* by Alison Hawthorne Deming (1994) in which the mass of the soul is estimated by weighing mice before and after they were chloroformed to death. The incongruity of the test is more fascinating than its predictive power.

Box 2.2 Probit concentration (or dose)–effect models: measuring precisely the wrong thing?

The first application of what eventually became the probit method was in the field of psychophysics. Soon thereafter, it was applied in mammalian toxicology to model quantal response data (e.g. dead or alive) generated from toxicity assays. Gaddum (as ascribed by Bliss and Cattell 1943) hypothesized an explanation for its application called alternately, the individual effective dose or individual tolerance hypothesis. Which name was used seemed to depend on whether the toxicant was administered as a dose or in some other way such as an exposure concentration. The concept was the same regardless of the exact name. Each individual was assumed to have an innate tolerance often expressed as an effective dose. The individual would survive if it received a dose below its effective dose but would die if its effective dose were reached or exceeded. Studies of drug or poison potencies conducted on individuals suggested that individual effective doses were log normally distributed in populations. This provided justification for fitting quantal data to a log normal (probit) model (Bliss 1935; Finney 1947; Gaddum 1953). For example, a common assay to determine the potency of a digitalis preparation was to slowly infuse an increasing dose of the preparation into individual cats until each one's heart just stopped beating. If enough cats were so treated, the distribution of effective doses would appear log normal.

Surprisingly, this central hypothesis has not been rigorously tested. The reason seems more historical than scientific. First, in the context of the early toxicity assays, the theory was discussed primarily to support the application of a log normal model. Second, it was easy to find genetic evidence of differences in tolerance among individuals. However, no studies defined the general magnitude of these differences among individuals in populations nor the rationale for why these differences should always be log normally distributed in populations. Third, the correctness of the theory was not as important in this context as in the one into which ecotoxicologists have thrust it.

Another explanation, already mentioned, exists and will be called the stochasticity hypothesis (Newman 1998; Newman and McCloskey 2000). Instead of a lethal dose being an innate characteristic of each individual, the risk of dying is the same for all individuals because the same stochastic processes are occurring in all individuals. Whether one or another individual dies at a particular dose is random with the resulting distribution of doses killing individuals described best by a log normal distribution. Gaddum (1953) described a random process involving several 'hits' at the site of action to cause death that resulted in a log normal distribution of deaths. Berkson (1951) describes an experiment supporting the stochastic theory. The experiment was done when he was hired as a consultant to analyze tolerances to high-altitude conditions of candidate aviators. Candidates were screened by being placed into a barometric chamber and then noting whether they fainted at high-altitude conditions. The premise was that those men with an inherently low tolerance to high-altitude conditions would be poor pilots. Berkson broke from the screening routine to challenge this individual tolerance concept. He asked that a group of pilots be retested to see if individuals retained their relative rankings between trials. They did not, indicating that the test and the individual effective dose concept were not valid in this case. In contrast, zebra fish (*Brachydanio rerio*) tolerance to the anesthetic, benzocaine, did more recently provide limited support for the individual effective dose concept (Newman and McCloskey 2000).

The crucial difference between these two models is whether the dose that actually kills or otherwise affects a particular individual is determined by an innate quality of the individual or by a random process taking place in all individuals. Determining under what conditions, which one or combination of these hypotheses is correct is important in determining the population consequences of exposure.

The importance of discerning between these two hypotheses can be illustrated with a simple thought experiment (Newman 1998). Assume that a concentration of exactly one LC50 results from a discharge into a stream for exactly 96 h. During the release, a population of similar individuals is exposed for 96 h to one LC50 and then to no toxicant for enough time to recover. For simplicity, we assume no post-exposure mortality. After ample time for recovery, the survivors in the population are exposed again. This process is repeated several times. Under the individual effective dose or individual tolerance hypothesis, 50% of the individuals would die during the first exposure. During any exposure thereafter, there would be no, or minimal, mortality because all survivors of the first exposure would have individual tolerances greater than the LC50. In contrast, the stochasticity hypothesis predicts a 50% loss of exposed individuals during each 96 h exposure. The population consequences are very different with these two hypotheses. In this thought experiment, the population remains extant (individual effective dose hypothesis) or eventually goes locally extinct (stochasticity hypothesis) (Figure 2.3). With some deliberation, the reader can likely find other situations in which it would be crucial to determine the appropriate theory in order to predict population fate under toxicant exposure.

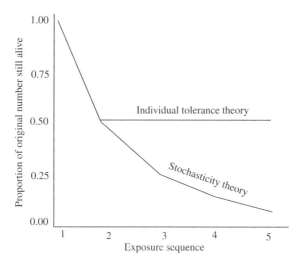

Fig. 2.3. The predicted decreases in size for a population receiving repeated exposures to one LC50 for exactly 96 h with ample time between exposures for recovery. Highly divergent outcomes are predicted based on the individual tolerance (individual effective dose) or stochasticity hypotheses. A blending of the two hypotheses (both processes are important in determining risk of death) would produce curves in the area between those for the individual tolerance and stochasticity theories

It would be surprising if the individual effective dose hypothesis were applicable to all or most ecotoxicity data to which the probit model is now applied. The probit method is applied to data for different effects under a variety of conditions to many species. It is applied to both clonal (e.g. *Daphnia magna* and *Vibrio fisheri*) and nonclonal collections of individuals. Nonclonal groups of individuals might be inbred, laboratory bred, or collected from the wild. It would be remarkable if the same explanation fits all diverse effects to such diverse collections of individuals. Indeed, recent work with sodium chloride toxicity to mosquitofish (*Gambusia holbrooki*) suggests that the individual effective dose concept is an inadequate explanation for all applications of the probit (log normal) model (Newman and McCloskey 2000).

Again, why has this ambiguity remained unresolved for so long? Because, following the lead of mammalian toxicologists, we have focused on the effects of toxicants on individuals and paid too little attention to translating effects metrics to population consequences.

2.3 INFERENCES WITHIN AND BETWEEN BIOLOGICAL LEVELS

In Chapter 1, several avenues for inference within and between biological levels were discussed. Microexplanation (reductionism) might be possible for population behavior based on the qualities of individuals. Acknowledging the unpredictable influence of emergent properties, a description (explanation without a strict knowledge of the underlying mechanism) might be made of a consistent response at the population level in a holistic study. Careful speculation from the population level to the level of the individual (macroexplanation) might be possible as long as the problem of ecological inference is acknowledged. Finally, one could project from the response of populations to the possible consequences to communities. Here, again, emergent properties might compromise predictions.

2.3.1 INFERRING POPULATION EFFECTS FROM QUALITIES OF INDIVIDUALS

Unquestionably, predicting population consequences from organismal and suborganismal effects is a major pursuit in ecotoxicology. Toxicant effects in individuals provide explanation for observed changes in field populations, e.g. DDT-induced changes in calcium-dependent ATPase in the egg-shell gland with consequent bird population failure (Kolaja and Hinton 1979). Subtle changes such as fluctuating asymmetry or developmental stability have potential as field indicators of contaminant influence on populations (Zakharov 1990; Graham, Freeman and Emlen 1993). Changes to individuals can imply changes in vital rates such as described for white sucker (*Catostomus commersoni*) in a metal-contaminated lake (McFarlane and Frazin 1978). Theoretical models for disease in populations (Moolgavkar 1986) and population impact of toxicants (Callow and Sibly 1990; Holloway, Sibley and Povenvan 1990) are also based on organismal and suborganismal information.

More and more frequently, vital rates derived from individuals in laboratory populations are applied to projections of population consequences of exposure (e.g. Postma, van Kleunen and Admiraal 1995; Pesch, Munns and Gutjahr-Gobell 1991). In some studies, problems associated with ecological inference can arise. For example, Pesch, Munns and Gutjahr-Gobell (1991) were required by the characteristics of their experimental species (the polychaete, *Neanthes arenaceo-dentata*) to derive fecundity and survival schedules from aggregated data instead of data from individuals.

2.3.2 INFERRING INDIVIDUAL EFFECTS FROM QUALITIES OF POPULATIONS

Inferences about individuals from population measurements (e.g. ecological inference) are sometimes desirable and yield meaningful knowledge if the problem of ecological inference is addressed carefully. This is the major difficulty of macroexplanation.

Surveys of genetic markers in toxicant-exposed populations exemplify inference about individuals based on population qualities. Allele frequencies determined for subsamples of populations inhabiting sites that differ in toxicant concentrations might be used to determine a relationship between allele frequency and exposure intensity (e.g. Sloss, Romano and Anderson 1998). The observation of such a statistically significant correlation often leads the investigator to argue that selection against certain genotypes occurred. Aggregate data (allele frequencies) are used to imply behavior of genotypes (individuals) as a consequence of exposure. However, alternate explanations exist such as toxicant-induced genetic bottlenecks or accelerated drift (Newman 1995). Genotype frequencies that are found to deviate significantly from Hardy–Weinberg expectations might be used to conclude that certain genotypes have lower fitnesses during exposure than others. However, other factors can produce departures from Hardy–Weinberg expectations including low population size, high migration rates, nonrandom breeding, and population structuring, i.e., the Wahlund effect seen by Woodward, Mulvey and Newman (1996). Although inferences from these types of data are important, without supporting experimentation on individuals, the problem of ecological inference precludes clear conclusions about individuals. Chapters 7 and 8 will cover these topics in population genetics in more detail.

Epidemiological studies often make inferences about individuals based on aggregated, population-level data. King (1997) gives the example of incorrectly predicting an individual's risk of dying of radon-induced lung cancer based on correlations between regional radon levels and fatal lung cancer rates. Without monitoring an individual's radon exposure for many years, ecological inference is the only recourse for the epidemiologist. Yet inferences about acceptable radon levels must be made by regulators without such extremely expensive information for radon exposure to individuals. As practical, assessment of human risk from air pollutants has slowly moved toward monitoring of individual exposures for this and other reasons, e.g. see Ryan's (1998) treatment of this topic. Because of constraints imposed by limited time and money, deriving plausible inferences about individual risk based on aggregated data will continue to be a major challenge in epidemiology, the subject of the next chapter.

2.3.3 INFERRING COMMUNITY EFFECTS FROM QUALITIES OF POPULATIONS

Inferences about communities from population or individual measurements are common but meaningful only if the question of emergent properties is addressed carefully. This is the general flaw of any attempt at microexplanation and can result in inaccurate prediction. For example, community structure can be indirectly changed by the removal of one keystone species, a species that influences the community by its activity or role, not its numerical dominance. Removal of sea urchins from a rocky intertidal pool results in a very dramatic shift in the composition of the epilithic algal species and biomass (Paine and Vadas 1969). A toxicant that kills urchins could produce a fundamental change in algal communities without having a direct effect on algal species. Field (Post, Frost and Kitchell 1995) and laboratory (Taylor *et al.* 1995) studies with freshwater invertebrates also suggest changes in community interactions (predator–prey relationships) as a consequence of toxicant exposure. Whether microexplanation would have predicted the importance of the interactions among populations based on community status is uncertain. Let's examine a regulatory practice that depends on individual-based knowledge (response of individuals in conventional toxicity tests) to imply the level of harm to an ecological community (Box 2.3).

Box 2.3   Protection of communities based on species NOEC values (Figure 2.4)

Most knowledge applied to setting effluent discharge limits or to ecological risk assessment comes from assays of toxicant effects on individuals, e.g. 96 h LC50, IC50, or NOEC. With some exceptions, the typical test involves exposure of groups of individuals to a series of toxicant concentrations for a predetermined time. A metric is derived based on such effects as the number of individuals dying, change in growth of exposed individuals, or change in reproductive output of exposed individuals. This preponderance of individual-based knowledge and the need to protect ecological communities have led to the application of individual-level test results to infer community consequences. As an important example, US numerical water-quality criteria have been based on 'an estimate of a concentration that will protect most but not all aquatic life; this concentration is defined as that which affects no more than 5% of taxa, with a proviso that important single species will also be protected' (Niederlehner *et al.* 1986). Although emergent properties can

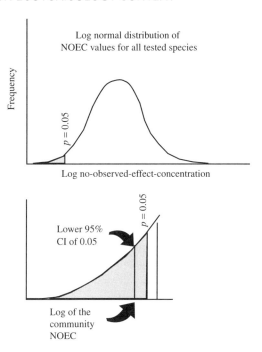

Fig. 2.4. Prediction of community NOEC (no-observed-effect-concentration) based on NOEC values for individual species notionally reflecting those in the community to be protected. The top panel is the log normal distribution of NOEC values for all tested species. The species are assumed to adequately represent those in an ecological community. The bottom panel depicts the derivation of a community NOEC or HCp from this distribution. One could select the NOEC value at $p = 5\%$ of species as the community NOEC. The assumption is that all but 5% of species in the community would be protected at this NOEC. A more conservative community NOEC can be established at the lower 95% tolerance limit of the 5% value

invalidate inferences of this sort, there are a few documented cases in which chronic effects to individuals did seem adequate for predicting community-level consequences, e.g. cadmium (Niederlehner *et al.* 1986) and diazinon (Giddings *et al.* 1996) in freshwater systems. Risk assessments are appearing based on this assumption that the distribution of effects metrics from single species tests allows adequate prediction of a concentration below which only an acceptable proportion of a community will be impacted. Provided keystone and dominant species are protected, redundancy in ecological communities may allow for a certain level of species loss before an adverse impact to the community occurs. Some recent examples of risk assessments based on this concept include estimations of risk associated with atrazine (a herbicide) use in North America (Solomon *et al.* 1996), and cadmium and copper in the Chesapeake Bay watershed (Hall, Scott and Killen 1998). This single-species test approach, growing out of regulatory necessity, was proposed in the mid-1980s. The uncertainty associated with extrapolation from acute, individual-based data for many species to ecosystem level effects was studied by Slooff Van Oers and De Zwart (1986). They produced a regression model predicting the log of the NOEC for a community from the log of the lowest LC50 or EC50 value from toxicity test data. The relationship had an r of 0.77, so roughly 59% (or r^2) of the variation in the log of NOEC for a community could be explained with the model. Considering that there was clearly scatter in these data and that log transformations of NOECs were being predicted, this suggests that prediction would be only grossly accurate. The authors recommended that a large uncertainty factor be employed to compensate in a conservative manner for this uncertainty. With this relationship and uncertainty factor, the authors concluded that acute toxicity information was useful for predicting 'ecosystem' effects.

It would have been useful to apply cross-validation methods to these data as this is the best way to actually estimate the predictive value of such a regression model. My own cross-validation analysis of their data using prediction sum of squares suggests that the overall predictive value of the regression model was acceptable. (See cross-validation procedures in statistical books such as Neter Wasserman and Kutner (1990), pp. 465–470 for more detail.)

Several changes have occurred in this general approach. Kooijman (1987) developed a log-logistic model for predicting the concentration affecting 5% of tested species (Figure 2.4, top drawing) and giving conditions under which this could be used for limited prediction of community protection. Kooijman (1987) also provided estimates of the optimum number of species needed to make predictions, basing these estimates on parametric methods. Kooijman was aware of the potential applications of his analyses and began his manuscript by stating,

The purpose of this paper is to define the concept of a hazardous concentration for sensitive species. . .[it] can be regarded as a lower bound for concentrations that can be expected to be harmful for a given community. . .
All honest scientific research workers will feel rather uncomfortable with such a task; and the author is no exception.

Van Straalen and Denneman (1989) extended this approach in risk-assessment activities to protect soil-dwelling organisms from contaminants. They modified Kooijman's mathematics to allow prediction of concentrations protecting all but a specified, low proportion of all species (p). Wagner and Løkke (1991) modified the approach further by fitting data to a log-normal instead of a log logistic model. More importantly, they suggested that the lower

95% tolerance limit of the predicted concentration affecting 5% of species be used as a conservative estimate of the hazardous concentration (HCp) (Figure 2.4, bottom drawing). Consequently, the hazardous concentration was fixed according to a specific level of confidence (expressed as a probability) in knowing that no more than a specified proportion of all species would be adversely affected. Wagner and Løkke (1991) specified that 95% of the time that such an analysis was done, no more than 5% of the species would be adversely affected at the calculated concentration. This compensates in a conservative direction for prediction uncertainty.

Considerable thought was put into the limitations of these methods as they began to be applied in regulations and assessments. Kooijman's original work (Kooijman 1987) and later comment by Hopkin (1993), Jagoe and Newman (1997), and Newman et al. (2000) focused on ecological and statistical limits to inference from this approach. The major concerns were summarized by Newman et al. (2000) as the following:

- LC50, EC50, NOEC and MATC data have significant deficiencies as measures of effect on natural populations. Any method based on extrapolation from these metrics shares their shortcomings.
- The assumption that redundancy in communities permits a certain proportion of species to be lost is based on the redundant species hypothesis. The alternate hypothesis, the rivet-popper hypothesis, suggests the opposite would be true and that any loss of species weakens a community. (See Pratt and Cairns 1996 for more detail.) Work with grassland communities lends some support to the rivet-popper hypothesis (Naeem et al. 1994; Tilman and Downing 1994; Tilman 1996; Tilman Wedlin and Knops 1996). Until ecologists determine which is the correct hypothesis, it would be best to be conservative and to adopt the rivet-popper context for regulatory action.
- The species-sensitivity distribution approach requires substantial knowledge of dominant and keystone species, and the importance of species interactions. Adequate knowledge is often not available to the ecotoxicologist. Also, even when important species and species interactions are considered, consideration is sometimes done short shrift.
- In situ exposure differs among species because of differences in their life histories, feeding habits, life stages, microhabitat, and other qualities. These differences are poorly reflected in the species-sensitivity distribution method because of the toxicity test design.
- There is a bias toward mortality data despite the likelihood of sublethal effects playing a crucial role in local extinction of exposed populations.
- A specific distribution, e.g. the log normal (probit) model, is assumed more out of tradition than careful consideration of alternatives. Newman et al (2000) and Jagoe and Newman (1997) demonstrated the inaccuracy of assuming such a model and advocated a bootstrap method for estimating

the HCp. The bootstrap method does not require a distribution to provide the HCp and associated confidence limits. Therefore, this particular shortcoming is easily resolvable.

• Determination of the optimum number of species required to produce a sound estimate of the HCp and the sample representativeness of the community to be protected are often given inadequate attention. However, the suboptimal sample size shortcoming can be resolved with more consistent application of parametric (Kooijman 1987) and nonparametric (Newman *et al.* 2000) methods for estimating optimum sample size.

These problems include technically resolvable issues and problems that can be characterized as ambiguities about emergent properties. Key to the use of this species-sensitivity distribution method to predict community-level consequences is thoughtfulness and caution based on an in-depth knowledge of the population qualities. Otherwise inference across two or more levels of organization is of questionable value and, at worst, is a source in false and distracting information. Gross approximations, e.g. implying species disappearance from a community based on a 96 h LC50, are forced on the ecotoxicologist as a regulatory necessity. Associated uncertainty must be dealt with by making estimates as conservative as reasonable.

2.4 SUMMARY

This chapter introduced the reader to population ecotoxicology, the science of contaminants in the biosphere and their effects on populations. Topics relevant to population ecotoxicology are epidemiology of toxicant-linked disease, basic demography, metapopulation biology, life history theory, and population genetics.

The need for exploring population ecotoxicology was defined in terms of its scientific and practical values. The emerging regulatory emphasis on predicting population consequences was contrasted with the preoccupation with generating information directly relevant to individuals.

Inferences within and between biological levels were explored from the perspective of the population. Application of individual and subindividual data to predict population consequences was described, emphasizing the importance of thoughtful awareness of emergent properties. Brief discussion of inferring individual behaviors based on population-level information demonstrated the problem of ecological inference, as well as the need for such inference. Epidemiology was identified as one relevant field in which such inferences occur. Finally, we discussed inferences based on individual- or population-level information to predict community fate upon toxicant exposure. A species-sensitivity distribution approach was used as an example. The problem of unforeseen emergent properties was again discussed as inhibiting clear inference about community effects from toxicity test results.

2.4.1 SUMMARY OF FOUNDATION CONCEPTS AND PARADIGMS

- Laws, regulations, and standards aim to protect the viability of natural populations in ecological communities. Consequently, population ecotoxicology has practical value.
- Effects to individuals measured in standard toxicity tests are intended for use in predicting consequences to exposed populations. They do this with ambiguous precision and accuracy.
- Classic studies in population biology and genetics involve response to toxicants. Consequently, population ecotoxicology has already demonstrated its scientific value.
- Inferences about individuals from population studies, e.g. some epidemiological studies, are valuable but prone to the problem of ecological inference.
- Inferences about communities from population studies are valuable but prone to error due to the emergence of unique properties at higher levels of biological organization.
- Inference based solely on an observed, consistent behavior of a population, often measured as a correlation, is valuable but prone to error because causal mechanisms are not defined. Knowledge of causation allows most accurate prediction under different conditions.
- Macroexplanation, microexplanation, and holism are most valuable and error-free if used together and with a full understanding of their shortcomings.

REFERENCES

Antonovics J, Bradshaw AD and Turner RG (1971). Heavy metal tolerance in plants. In *Advances in Ecological Research Vol. 7*, ed. by JB Cragg, pp. 1–83. Academic Press, London.

Asami T and Grant B (1994). Melanism has not evolved in Japanese *Biston betularia* (Geometridae). *J Lepid Soc* **49**: 88–91.

Barnthouse LW, Suter II GW, Rosen AE and Beauchamp JJ (1987). Estimating responses of fish populations to toxic contaminants. *Environ Toxicol Chem* **6**: 811–824.

Beardmore JA (1980). Genetical considerations in monitoring effects of pollution. *Rapp P-v Réun Cons Int Explor Mer* **179**: 258–266.

Beaumont P (1997). Where have all the birds gone? *Pesticides News* **30**: 3.

Berkson J (1951). Why I prefer logits to probits. *Biometrics* **7**: 327–339.

Berry RJ (1990). Industrial melanism and peppered moths (*Biston betularia* (L.)). *Biol J Linn Soc* **39**: 301–322.

Bishop JA and Hartley DJ (1976). The size and structure of rural populations of*Rattus norvegicus* containing individuals resistant to the anticoagulant poison Warfarin. *J Anim Ecol* **45**: 623–646.

Bishop JA, Hartley DJ and Partridge GG (1977). The population dynamics of genetically determined resistance to Warfarin in *Rattus norvegicus* from mid-Wales. *Heredity* **39**: 389–398.

Bliss CI (1935). The calculation of the dosage–mortality curve. *Ann Appl Biol* **22**: 134–307.

Bliss CI and Cattell M (1943). Biological assay. *Ann Rev Physiol* **5**: 479–539.

Boyd CE and Ferguson DE (1964). Susceptibility and resistance of mosquito fish to several insecticides. *J Economic Entomol* **57**: 430–431.

Brakefield PM (1990). A decline of melanism in the peppered moth *Biston betularia* in The Netherlands. *Biol J Linn Soc* **39**: 327–334.

Brown JH and Maurer BA (1989). Macroecology: the division of food and space among species on continents. *Science* **243**: 1145–1150.

Cairns, Jr J and Pratt JR (1989). The scientific basis of bioassays. *Hydrobiologia* **188/189**: 5–20.

Calow P and Sibly RM (1990). A physiological basis of population processes: ecotoxicological implications. *Funct Ecol* **4**: 283–288.

Carson R (1962). *Silent Spring*. Houghton-Mifflin, Boston, MA.

Caswell H (1996). Demography meets ecotoxicology: untangling the population level effects of toxic substances. In *Ecotoxicology. A Hierarchical Treatment* ed. by MC Newman and CH Jagoe, pp. 255–292. CRC/Lewis Press, Boca Raton, FL.

Clarke CA, Grant B, Clarke FMM and Asami T (1994). A long term assessment of *Biston betularis* (L.) in one U.K. locality (Caldy Common near Kirby, Wirral), 1959–1993, and glimpses elsewhere. *The Linnean* **10**: 18–26.

Clarke CA, Mani GS and Wynne G (1985). Evolution in reverse: clean air and the peppered moth. *Biol J Linn Soc* **26**: 189–199.

Comins HN (1977). The development of insecticide resistance in the presence of migration. *J Theor Biol* **64**: 177–197.

Connell DW and Miller DJ (1984). *Chemistry and Ecotoxicology of Pollution*. John Wiley, New York.

Deming AH (1994). *Science and Other Poems*. Louisiana State University Press, Baton Rouge, LA.

Dixon PM and Newman MC (1991). Analyzing toxicity data using statistical models of time-to-death: an introduction. In *Metal Ecotoxicology. Concepts & Application*, ed. by MC Newman and AW McIntosh, pp. 207–242. CRC/Lewis Press, Chelsea, MI.

Dolphin R (1959). Lake County mosquito abatement district gnat research program. Clear Lake Gnat (*Chaoborus astictopus*). Proceedings of 27th Annual Conference of the California Mosquito Control Association, pp. 47–48.

Emlen JM (1989). Terrestrial population models for ecological risk assessment: A state-of-the-art review. *Environ Toxicol Chem* **8**: 831–842.

EPA (1991). Summary Report on Issues in Ecological Risk Assessment, EPA/625/3–91/018, February. NTIS, Springfield, VA.

Finney DJ (1947). *Probit Analysis. A Statistical Treatment of the Sigmoid Response Curve*. Cambridge University Press, Cambridge.

Forbes VE and Forbes TL (1994). Ecotoxicology in Theory and Practice. Chapman and Hall, London.

Fry DM and Toone CK (1981). DDT-induced feminization of gull embryos. *Science* **213**: 922–924.

Gaddum JH (1953). Bioassays and mathematics. *Pharmacol Rev* **5**: 87–134.

Giddings JM, Biever RC, Annunziato MF, and Hosmer AJ (1996). Effects of diazinon on large outdoor pond microcosms. *Environ Toxicol Chem* **15**: 618–629.

Ginzburg LR, Johnson K, Pugliese A and Gladden J (1984). Ecological risk assessment based on stochastic age-structure models of population growth. In *Statistics in the*

Environmental Sciences, ASTM STP 845 ed. by SM Gertz and MD London pp. 31–45. American Society for Testing and Materials, Philadelphia, PA.

Graham JH, Freeman DC, and Emlen JM (1993). Developmental stability: a sensitive indicator of populations under stress. In *Environmental Toxicology and Risk Assessment, ASTM STP 1179*, ed. by WG Landis, JS, Hughes and MA Lewis pp. 136–158, American Society for Testing and Materials, Philadelphia, PA.

Grant BS and Howlett RJ (1988). Background selection by the peppered moth (*Biston betularia* Linn.): individual differences. *Biol J Linn Soc* **33**: 217–232.

Grant BS, Clarke CA, (1999). An examination of intraseasonal variation in the incidence of melanism in peppered moths, **Biston betularia**. *J. Lepid Soc* **53**: 99–103.

Grant BS, Cook AD, Clarke CA and Owen DF (1998). Geographic and temporal variation in the incidence of melanism in peppered moth populations in America and Britain. *J Hered* **89**: 465–471.

Grant BS, Owen DF, and Clarke CA (1995). Decline of melanic moths. *Nature* **373**: 565.

Grant BS, Owen DF, and Clare CA (1996). Parallel rise and fall of melanic peppered moths in America and Britain. *J Hered* **87**: 351–357.

Green AS and Chandler GT (1996). Life-table evaluation of sediment-associated chlorpyrifos chronic toxicity to the benthic copepod, *Amphiascus tenuiremis*. *Arch Environ Contam Toxicol* **31**: 77–83.

Guttman SI (1994). Population genetic structure and ecotoxicology. *Environ Health Perspect* **102**(Suppl. 12):97–100.

Hall Jr LW, Scott MC, and Killen WD (1998). Ecological risk assessment of copper and cadmium in surface waters of Chesapeake Bay watershed. *Environ Toxicol Chem* **17**: 1172–1189.

Hickey JJ and Anderson DW (1968). Chlorinated hydrocarbons and eggshell changes in raptorial and fish-eating birds. *Science* **162**: 271–273.

Hopkin SP (1993). Ecological implications of '95% protection levels' for metals in soil. *OIKOS* **66**: 137–141.

Holloway GJ, Sibly RM, and Povey SR (1990). Evolution in toxin-stressed environments. *Functional Ecol* **4**: 289–294.

Jagoe RH and Newman MC (1997). Bootstrap estimation of community NOEC values. *Ecotoxicology* **6**: 293–306.

Kammenga JE, Busschers M, Van Straalen NM, Jepson PC, and Baker J (1996). Stress induced fitness is not determined by the most sensitive life-cycle trait. *Functional Ecol* **10**: 106–111.

Karås P, Neuman E, and Sandström O (1991). Effects of a pulp mill effluent on the population dynamics of perch, *Perca fluviatilis*. *Can J Fish Aquat Sci* **48**: 28–34.

Kettlewell HBD (1955). Selection experiments on industrial melanism in the Lepidoptera. *Heredity* **9**: 323–342.

Kettlewell HBD (1973). The Evolution of Melanism. Claredon Press, Oxford.

King G (1997). A Solution to the Ecological Inference Problem. Princeton University Press, Princeton, NJ.

Klerks PL and Weis JS (1987). Genetic adaptation to heavy metals in aquatic organisms: A review. *Environ Pollut* **45**: 173–205.

Kolaja GJ and Hinton DE (1979). *Animals as Monitors of Environmental Pollutants*, pp. 309–318. National Academy of Sciences, Washington, DC.

Kooijman SALM (1987). A safety factor for LC_{50} values allowing for differences in sensitivity among species. *Wat Res* **21**: 269–276.

Landis WG and Yu M-H (1995). *Introduction to Environmental Toxicology: Impacts of Chemicals upon Ecological Systems*. CRC Press, Boca Raton, FL.

Lee DR and Creed ER (1977). The genetics of the *insularia* forms of the peppered moth, *Biston betularia*. *J Anim Ecol* **39**: 67–73.

Luoma JR (1992). New effect of pollutants: Hormone mayhem. *New York Times*, 24 May.

Maciorowski AF (1988). Populations and communities: linking toxicology and ecology in a new synthesis. *Environ Toxicol Chem* **7**: 677–678.

Mani GS (1990). Theoretical models of melanism in *Biston betularia* — a review. *Biol J Linn Soc* **39**: 355–371.

McFarlane GA and Franzin WG (1978). Elevated heavy metals: a stress on a population of white suckers, *Catostomus commersoni*, in Hamell Lake, Saskatchewan. *J Fish Res Board Can* **35**: 963–970.

McKenzie JA and Batterham P (1994). The genetic, molecular and phenotypic consequences of selection for insecticide resistance. *TREE* **9**: 166–169.

McLachlan JA (1993). Functional toxicology: A new approach to detect biologically active xenobiotics. *Environ Health Perspect* **101**: 386–387.

Mitton JB (1997). *Selection in Natural Populations*. Oxford University Press, Oxford.

Moolgavkar SH (1986). Carcinogenesis modeling: from molecular biology to epidemiology. *Ann Rev Public Health* **7**: 151–169.

Mulvey M and Diamond SA (1991). Genetic factors and tolerance acquisition in populations exposed to metals and metalloids. In *Metal Ecotoxicology. Concepts & Applications*, ed. by MC Newman and AW McIntosh, pp. 301–321. CRC/Lewis Press, Chelsea, MI.

Mulvey M, Newman MC, Chazal A, Keklak MM, Heagler HG and Hales S (1995). Genetic and demographic changes in mosquitofish (*Gambusia holbrooki*) populations exposed to mercury. *Environ Toxicol Chem* **14**: 1411–1418.

Naeem S, Thompson LJ, Lawler SP, Lawton JH, and Woodfin RM (1994). Declining biodiversity can alter performance of ecosystems. *Nature* **368**: 734–737.

Neter J, Wasserman W and Kutner WH (1990). *Applied Linear Statistical Models. Regression, Analysis of Variance, and Experimental Design*. Richard D. Irwin, Homewood, IL.

Newman MC (1995). *Quantitative Methods in Aquatic Ecotoxicology*. CRC/Lewis Press, Boca Raton, FL.

Newman MC (1998). *Fundamentals of Ecotoxicology*. CRC/Ann Arbor Press, Boca Raton, FL.

Newman MC and Aplin M (1992). Enhancing toxicity data interpretation and prediction of ecological risk with survival time modeling: an illustration using sodium chloride toxicity to mosquitofish (*Gambusia holbrooki*). *Aquat Toxicol* **23**: 85–96.

Newman MC and Dixon PM (1996). Ecologically meaningful estimates of lethal effect on individuals. In *Ecotoxicology: A Hierarchical Treatment*, ed. by MC Newman and CH Jagoe, pp. 225–253. Boca Raton, FL: CRC/Lewis Press.

Newman MC and McCloskey JT (1996). Time-to-event analysis of ectotoxicity data.*Ecotoxicology* **5**: 187–196.

Newman MC and McCloskey JT (2000). The individual tolerance concept is not the sole explanation for the probit dose–effect model. *Environ Toxicol Chem* **19**: 520–526.

Newman MC, Ownby DR, Mézin LCA, Powell DC, Christensen TRL, Lerberg SB, and Anderson B-A. (2000). Applying species sensitivity distributions in ecological risk assessment: assumptions of distribution type and sufficient numbers of species. *Environ Toxicol Chem* **19**: 508–515.

Niederlehner BR, Pratt JR, Buikema Jr AL and Cairns Jr J (1986). Comparison of estimates of hazard derived at three levels of complexity. In *Community Toxicity Testing, ASTM STP 920*, ed. by J. Cairns Jr, pp. 30–48. American Society for Testing and Materials, Philadelphia, PA.

O'Connor RJ (1996). Toward the incorporation of spatiotemporal dynamics in ecotoxicology. In *Population Dynamics in Ecological Space and Time*, ed. by OE Rhodes Jr, RK Chesser and MH Smith, pp. 281–317. University of Chicago Press, Chicago, IL.

Odum EP (1971). *Fundamentals of Ecology*, (3rd edn). W.B. Saunders Co., Philadelphia, PA.

Osowski SL, Brewer LW, Baker OE, and Cobb GP (1995). The decline of mink in Georgia, North Carolina, and South Carolina: the role of contaminants. *Arch Environ Contam Toxicol* **29**: 418–423.

Paine RT and Vadas RL (1969). The effects of grazing by sea urchins, *Strongylocentrotus spp.*, on benthic algal populations. *Limnol Oceanogr* **14**: 710–719.

Parrish PR (1985). Acute toxicity tests. In *Fundamentals of Aquatic Toxicology*, ed. by GM Rand and SR Petrocelli pp. 31–57. Hemisphere Publishing Corp., Washington, DC.

Pesch CE, Munns Jr WR and Gutjahr-Gobell R (1991). Effects of a contaminated sediment on life history traits and population growth rate of *Neanthes arenaceodentata* (Polychaeta: Nereidae) in the laboratory. *Environ Toxicol Chem* **10**: 805–815.

Petersen Jr RC and Petersen LB-M. (1988). Compensatory mortality in aquatic populations: its importance for interpretation of toxicant effects. *Ambio* **17**: 381–386.

Post DM, Frost TM, and Kitchell JF (1995). Morphological responses by *Bosmina longirostris* and *Eubosmina tubicen* to changes in copepod predator populations during a whole-lake acidification experiment. *J Plankton Res* **17**: 1621–1632.

Postma JF, van Kleunen A, and Admiraal W (1995). Alterations in life-history traits of *Chironomus riparius* (Diptera) obtained from metal contaminated rivers. *Arch Environ Contam Toxicol* **29**: 469–475.

Pratt JR and Cairns Jr J (1996). Ecotoxicology and the redundancy problem: understanding effects on community structure and function. In *Ecotoxicology. A Hierarchical Treatment*, ed. by MC Newman and CH Jagoe pp. 347–370. CRC/Lewis Press, Boca Raton, FL.

Ratcliffe DA (1967). Decrease in eggshell weight in certain birds of prey. *Nature* **215**: 208–210.

Ratcliffe DA (1970). Changes attributable to pesticides in egg breakage frequency and eggshell thickness in some British birds. *J Appl Ecol* **7**: 67–107.

Ryan PB (1998). Historical perspective on the role of exposure assessment in human risk assessment. In *Risk Assessment: Logic and Measurement*, ed. by MC Newman and CL Strojan, pp. 23–43. Ann Arbor Press, Chelsea, MI.

Sarokin D and Schulkin J (1992). The role of pollution in large-scale population disturbances. Part 1: aquatic populations. *Environ Sci Technol* **26**: 1476–1484.

Sierszen ME and Frost TM (1993). Response of predatory zooplankton populations to the experimental acidification of Little Rock Lake, Wisconsin. *J Plankton Res* **15**: 553–562.

Slooff W, Van Oers JAM., and De Zwart D (1986). Margins of uncertainty in ecotoxicological hazard assessment. *Environ Toxicol Chem* **5**: 841–852.

Sloss BL, Romano MA, and Anderson RV (1998). Pollution-tolerant allele in fingernail clams (*Musculium transversum*). *Arch Environ Contam Toxicol* **35**: 302–308.

Solomon KR, Baker DB, Richards RP, Dixon KR, Klaine SJ, La Point TW, Kendall RJ, Weisskopf CP, Giddings JM, Giesy JP, Hall Jr LW and Williams WM (1996). Ecological risk assessment of atrazine in North American surface waters. *Environ Toxicol Chem* **15**: 31–76.

Spitzer PR, Risebrough RW, Walker, II W, Hernandez R, Poole A, Puleston D, and Nisbet ICT (1978). Productivity of ospreys in Connecticut-Long Island increase as DDE residues decline. *Science* **202**: 333–335.

Suter, II GW (1993). *Ecological Risk Assessment*. Lewis Publishers, Chelsea, MI.

Taylor EJ, Morrison JE, Blockwell SJ, Tarr A, and Pascoe D (1995). Effects of lindane on the predator–prey interaction between *Hydra oligactis* Pallas and *Daphnia magna* Strauss. *Arch Environ Contam Toxicol* **29**: 291–296.

Tilman D (1996). Biodiversity: population versus ecosystem stability. *Ecology* **77**: 350–363.
Tilman D and Downing JA (1994). Biodiversity and stability on grasslands. *Nature* **367**: 363–365.
Tilman D, Wedlin D and Knops J (1996). Productivity and sustainability influenced by biodiversity in grassland ecosystems. *Nature* **379**: 718–720.
Trevan JW (1927). The error of determinations of toxicity. *Proc R Soc Lond B Biol Sci* **101**: 483–514.
Van Straalen NM and Denneman CAJ. (1989). Ecotoxicological evaluation of soil quality criteria. *Ecotox Environ Safety* **18**: 241–251.
Wagner C and Løkke H (1991). Estimation of ecotoxicological protection levels from NOEC toxicity data. *Wat Res* **25**: 1237–1242.
Wake DB (1991). Declining amphibian populations. *Science* **253**: 860.
Webb RE and Horsfall Jr F. (1967). Endrin resistance in the pine mouse. *Science* **156**: 1762.
Weis JS and Weis P (1989). Tolerance and stress in a polluted environment. *BioScience* **39**: 89–95.
West DA (1977). Melanism in *Biston* (Lepidoptera: Geometridae) in the rural Central Appalachians. *Heredity* **39**: 75–81.
Whitton MJ, Dearn JM, and McKenzie JA (1980). Field studies on insecticide resistance in the Australian sheep blowfly, *Lucilia cuprina*. *Aust J Biol* **33**: 725–735.
Woodward LA, Mulvey M and Newman MC (1996). Mercury contamination and population-level responses in chironomids: can allozyme polymorphisms indicate exposure? *Environ Toxicol Chem* **15**: 1309–1316.
Woodwell GM, Wurster Jr CF and Isaacson PA (1967). DDT residues in an East Coast estuary: a case of biological concentration of a persistent insecticide. *Science* **156**: 821–823.
Zakharov VM (1990). Analysis of fluctuating asymmetry as a method of biomonitoring at the population level. In *Bioindicators of Chemical and Radioactive Pollution*, ed. by DA Krivolutsky pp. 187–198. CRC Press, Boca Raton, FL.

3 Epidemiology: The Study of Disease in Populations

All scientific work is incomplete—whether it be observational or experimental. All scientific work is liable to be upset or modified by advancing knowledge. That does not confer upon us a freedom to ignore the knowledge we already have, or to postpone the action that it appears to demand at a given time. (Hill 1965)

3.1 FOUNDATION CONCEPTS AND METRICS IN EPIDEMIOLOGY

In environmental toxicology, methods may be applied to populations with two different purposes. The goal may be protection of either individuals or an entire population. This distinction is often confused in ecotoxicology, a science that must consider many levels of biological organization in its deliberations.

When dealing with contamination-associated disease in human populations, information is collected to protect individuals with certain characteristics such as high exposure or hypersensitivity. The emphasis is on identifying causal and etiological factors that put one individual at higher risk than another, and quantifying the likelihood of the disease afflicting an individual characterized relative to these risk factors. In contrast, in the study of nonhuman species, the focus shifts more toward maintaining viable populations than toward minimizing risk to specific individuals. Important exceptions involve the protection of endangered, threatened, or particularly charismatic species. In such cases, individuals may be the protected entities.

The focus in this chapter will be on epidemiology, the science concerned with the cause, incidence, prevalence, and distribution of disease in populations. More specifically, we will emphasize ecological epidemiology, that is, epidemiological methods applied to assess risk to nonhuman species inhabiting contaminated sites (Suter 1993). Methods described will provide insights of direct use for protecting individuals and describing disease presence in populations, and of indirect use for implying population consequences.

3.1.1 FOUNDATION CONCEPTS
In the above paragraph describing epidemiology, mention was made without explanation of causal and etiological factors. Let's take a moment to explain these terms and some associated concepts.

A causal agent is that causing something to occur directly or indirectly through a chain of events. Although seemingly obvious, this definition carries many philo sophical and practical complications.

Causation, a change in state or condition of one thing due to interaction with another, is surprisingly difficult to identify. One can identify a cause by applying the push-mechanism context of Descartes (Popper 1965) or Kant's (1934) concept of action. In this context, some cause has an innate power to produce an effect and is connected with that effect (Harré 1972). As an example, one body might pull (via gravity) or push (via magnetism) another by existing relative to that other. This results in motion. The presence and nature of the object cause a consequence and the effect diminishes with distance between the objects.

Alternatively, a cause may be defined in the context of succession theory as something preceding a specific event or change in state (Harré 1972). Kant (1934) refers to this as the Law of Succession in Time. The consistent sequence of one event (e.g. high exposure to a toxicant) followed by another (e.g. death) establishes an expectation. Based on past observations or observations reported by others, one comes to expect death after exposure to high concentrations of the toxicant.

Building from the thoughts of Popper (1959) regarding qualities of scientific inquiry, other qualities associated with the concept of causation emerge. Often there is an experimental design within which an effect is measured after a single thing is varied, i.e. the potential cause. The design of the experiment in which one thing is selected to be changed determines directly the context in which the term, cause, is applied. That which was varied causes the effect, e.g. increasing temperature caused an increase in bacterial growth rate. If another factor (e.g. an essential nutrient) had been varied in the experiment, it could have also caused the effect (e.g. increased growth rate). The following quote by Simkiss (1996) illustrates the importance of context and training in formulating causal structures.

> Thus, the problem took the form of habitat pollution ⟶ DDE accumulated in prey species ⟶ DDE in predators ⟶ decline in brood size ⟶ potential extermination. The same phenomenon can, however, be written in a different form. Lipid soluble toxicant ⟶ bioaccumulation in organisms with poor detoxification systems (birds metabolize DDE very poorly when compared with mammals) ⟶ vulnerable target organs (i.e., the shell gland has a high Ca flux) ⟶ inhibition of membrane-bound ATPases at crucial periods ⟶ potential extermination. Ecologists would claim a decline in population recruitment, biochemists an inhibition of membrane enzymes.

Clearly the context of observations and experiments, and measured parameters determined the causal structure for the ecologist (i.e. DDE spraying causes bird population extinctions) and biochemist (i.e. DDE bioaccumulation causes shell gland ATPase inhibition) studying the same phenomenon.

Controlled laboratory experiments remain invaluable tools for assigning causation as long as one understands the conditional nature of associated results. A co-existence of potential cause and effect is imposed unambiguously by the experimental design (Kant 1934), e.g. death occurred after 24 h exposure to

2 µg/L of dissolved toxicant in surrounding water. With this unambiguous co-occurrence and simplicity (low dimensionality), a high degree of consistency is expected from structured experiments. Also, one is capable of easily falsifying the hypothesized cause–effect relationship during structured experimentation. Inferences about causation are strengthened by these qualities of experiments. Information on causal linkage emerging from such a context is invaluable in ecological epidemiology but it is not the only type of useful information. Equally valuable information is obtained from less structured, observational 'experiments' possessing a lower ability to identify causal structure. Epidemiology relies heavily on such observational information.

Other factors complicate the process by which we effectively identify a cause–effect relationship in a world filled with interactions and change. According to Kant (1934), our minds are designed to create or impose useful structures of expectation that are not necessarily as grounded in objective reality as we might want to believe. We survive by developing webs of expectations based on unstructured observations of the world and by then pragmatically assigning causation within this complex. With incomplete knowledge and increasing complexity (high dimensionality), we often are compelled to build causal hypotheses from correlations (a probabilistic expectation based on past experience that depends heavily on the Law of Succession) and presumed mechanisms (linked cause–effect relationships leaning heavily on the concept of action). This is the wobbly foundation of everyday 'common sense', the expert opinion approach in ecological risk assessment, and pseudo-reasoning in cognitive studies. Unfortunately, habits applied in our informal reasoning are remarkably bad at determining the likelihood of one factor being a cause of a consequence if several candidate causes exist. Piattelli-Palmarini (1994) concluded that when we use our natural mental economy, '...we are *instinctively* very poor evaluators of probability and equally poor at choosing between alternative possibilities'. It follows from this sobering conclusion that accurate assignment of causation in ecotoxicology can more readily be made by formal methods, e.g. Bayesian logic, than by informal expert opinions and weight-of-evidence methods. This is especially important to keep in mind in ecological epidemiology.

These aspects of causation can be summarized in the points below. They provide context for judging the strength of inferences about causal agents from epidemiological studies.

- Causation is most commonly framed within the concept of action and the Law of Succession.
- Causation emerges as much from our 'neither rational nor capricious' (Tversky and Kahneman 1992) cognitive psychology as from objective reality.
- Causal structure emerges from an experimental framework as well as objective reality.

• Accurate identification of causation is enhanced by (1) clear co-occurrence in appropriate proximity of cause and effect, (2) simplicity (low dimensionality) of the system being assessed, (3) high degree of consistency from the system under scrutiny, and (4) formalization of the process for identifying causation.

Many of the conditions required to best identify causation are frequently absent in epidemiological studies. Therefore, when assessing effects of environmental contaminants, we resort to an assortment of correlative and mechanistic (cause–effect) information. Uncertainty about cause–effect linkages tempers terminology and forces logical qualifiers on conclusions. For example, a contaminant might be defined as an etiological agent, that is, something causing, initiating, or promoting disease. Notice that an etiological agent needn't be proven to be the causal agent. Indeed, with the multiple causation structure present in the real world and the compulsion of humans to construct subjective cause–effect relationships, the context of etiological agent seems more reasonable at times than that of causal agent.

Often epidemiology focuses on qualities of individuals that predispose them to some adverse consequence. In the context of cause–effect, such a factor is seen more as contributing to risk than as the direct cause of the effect. Such risk factors for human disease include genetic qualities of individuals, behaviors, diet, and exercise habitats. The presence of a benthic stage in the life cycle of an aquatic species might be viewed as a predisposing risk factor for the effects of a contaminant found in sediments. Possession of a gizzard in which swallowed 'stones' are ground together under acidic conditions could be considered a risk factor for lead poisoning of ducks dabbling in marshes spattered with lead shot from a nearby skeet range.

Clarification of the terms, risk and hazard, is necessary at this point. Hazard and risk are not synonymous terms in ecological epidemiology. The general meaning of risk is a danger or hazard, or the chance of something adverse happening. This is close to the definition that we will use. Hazard is defined here as simply the presence of a potential danger. For example, the hazard associated with a chemical may be grossly assessed by dividing its measured concentration in the environment by a concentration shown in the laboratory to cause an adverse effect. A hazard quotient exceeding one implies a potentially hazardous concentration. (Note that hazard will be defined differently when survival time modeling is discussed later in this chapter.) The concept of risk implies more than the presence of a potential danger. Risk is the probability of a particular adverse consequence occurring due to the presence of a causal agent, etiological agent, or risk factor. The concept of risk involves not only the presence of a danger but also the probability of the adverse effect being expressed in the population when the agent is present (Suter 1993).

Although defined as a probability, the concept of risk may be conveyed in other ways such as loss in life expectancy, e.g. a loss of 870 days from the average life span due to chronic exposure to a toxicant in the work environment. In the context of comparing populations or groups, it could be expressed as a relative risk, e.g. the risk of death at a 1 mg dose versus the risk of death at a 5 mg dose. It can also be expressed as an odds ratio or as an incidence rate. These metrics are defined in more detail below.

3.1.2 FOUNDATION METRICS

There are several straightforward metrics used in epidemiological analyses. Here, they will be discussed primarily in a human context but they are readily applied to nonhuman species. In fact, because of ethical limits on human experimentation, some metrics such as those generated from case–control or dose–effect studies are much more easily derived for nonhuman species than for humans.

Disease incidence rate for a nonfatal condition is measured as the number of individuals with the disease (N) divided by the total time that the population has been exposed (T). Incidence rate (I) is expressed in units of individuals or cases per unit of exposure time being considered in the study, e.g. 10 new cases per 1000 person-years (Ahlbom 1993). The T is expressed as the total number of time units that individuals were at risk, e.g. per 1000 person-years of exposure:

$$\hat{I} = \frac{N}{T} \qquad (3.1)$$

The number of individuals with the disease (N) is assumed to fit a Poisson distribution because a binomial error process is involved: an individual either does or does not have the disease. Consequently, the estimated mean of N is also an estimate of its variance. Knowing the variance of N, its 95% confidence limits can be estimated. Then, the 95% confidence limits of I can be estimated by dividing the upper and lower limits for N by T.

There are several ways of estimating the 95% confidence limits of N. Approximation under the assumption of a normal distribution instead of a Poisson distribution produces the following estimate (Ahlbom 1993):

$$\text{Number of cases} \approx \hat{N} \pm 1.96\sqrt{\hat{N}} \qquad (3.2)$$

To get the 95% confidence limits for I, those for N are divided by T. This and the other normal approximations described below can be poor estimators if the number of disease cases is small. The reader is referred to Ahlbom (1993) and Sahai and Khurshid (1996) for necessary details for such cases.

Estimated disease prevalence (P) is the incidence rate (I) times the length of time (t) that individuals were at risk:

$$\hat{P} = \hat{I} \times t \qquad (3.3)$$

For example, if there were 27 cases per 1000 person-years, the prevalence in a population of 10 000 people exposed for 10 years (i.e. 100 000 person-years) would be (27 cases/1000 person years)(100 000 person-years) or 2700 cases. Prevalence also emerges from a binomial error process, and its variance and confidence limits can be approximated as described above for incidence rate (Ahlbom 1993).

Sometimes it is advantageous to express the occurrence of disease in a population relative to that in another: often one population is a reference population. Differences in incidence rates can be used. For example, there may be 227 more cases per year in population A than in population B. Differences are often normalized to a specific population size (e.g. 227 more cases per year in a population of 10 000 individuals) because populations will differ in size.

Let's demonstrate the estimation of incidence rate difference and its confidence limits by considering two populations with person-exposure times of T_1 and T_2, and case numbers of N_1 and N_2 during those person-year intervals. The incidence rate difference (IRD) is estimated by the simple relationship,

$$\hat{IRD} = \frac{N_1}{T_1} - \frac{N_2}{T_2} \qquad (3.4)$$

The variance and confidence limits for the incidence rate difference are approximated by equations (3.5) and (3.6), respectively (Sahai and Khurshid 1996):

$$\text{Variance of } \hat{IRD} = \frac{N_1}{T_1^2} + \frac{N_2}{T_2^2} \qquad (3.5)$$

$$\hat{IRD} \pm Z_{\alpha/2} \sqrt{\frac{N_1}{T_1^2} + \frac{N_2}{T_2^2}} \qquad (3.6)$$

These equations can be applied during surveys of two populations or to case–control studies. N_1 and T_1 could be associated with one population and N_2 and T_2 with another. Or N_1 and T_1 could reflect the disease incidence rate for N_1 individuals known to have been exposed to an etiological agent, and N_2 and T_2 could reflect the effect incidence rate for N_2 individuals with no known exposure to the etiological agent. Individuals designated as a control or noncase group are compared to a group known to have been exposed in such retrospective case–control studies. The magnitude of the IRD suggests the influence of the etiological factor on the disease incidence.

The relative occurrence of disease in two populations can be expressed as the ratio of incidence rates (rate ratio). Equation (3.7) provides an estimate of the rate ratio for two populations:

$$\hat{RR} = \frac{\hat{I}_1}{\hat{I}_0} \qquad (3.7)$$

where $I_1 = $ incidence rate in population 1, and $I_0 = $ incidence rate in the reference or control population. For example, 20 diseased fish appearing annually in a standard sample size of 10 000 individuals taken from a bay near a heavily industrialized city may be compared to an annual incidence rate of 5 fish per 10 000 individuals from a bay adjacent to a small town. The relative risk in these populations would be estimated with a rate ratio of 4. Implied by this ratio is an influence of heavy industry on the risk of disease in populations. Obviously, an estimate of the variation about this ratio would contribute to a more definitive statement.

The variance and confidence limits for incidence rate ratios are usually derived in the context of the ln of rate ratios. The approximate variance and 95% confidence limits for the ln of rate ratio are defined by equations (3.8) and (3.9). The antilogarithm of the confidence limits approximate those for the rate ratio (Sahai and Khurshid 1996).

$$\text{Variance of } \ln\ (RR) \approx \frac{1}{N_1} + \frac{1}{N_0} \tag{3.8}$$

$$\ln RR \pm Z_{\alpha/2}\sqrt{\frac{1}{N_1} + \frac{1}{N_0}} \tag{3.9}$$

Box 3.1   Differences and ratios as measures of human risk

Cancer incidence rate differences at Love Canal

The building of the Love Canal housing tract around an abandoned waste burial site in New York resulted in one of the most public and controversial of human risk assessments. Approximately 21 800 tons of chemical waste were buried there starting in the 1920s and ending in 1953. Then housing units in the area increased rapidly, with 4897 people living on the tract by 1970. Public concern about the waste became acute in 1978. Enormous amounts of emotion and resources were justifiably expended trying to determine the risk to residents due to their close proximity to the buried waste. Based on chromosomal aberration data, the 1980 Picciano pilot study suggested that residents might be at risk of cancer but the results were not definitive. Ambiguity arose because of a lack of controls and disagreement about extrapolation from chromosomal aberrations to cancer and birth defects (Culliton 1980). Benzene and chlorinated solvents that were known or suspected to be carcinogens were present in the waste. However, extensive chemical monitoring by EPA suggested that the general area was safe for habitation and only a narrow region near the buried waste was significantly contaminated (Smith 1982a,b).

Because of their mode of action and toxicokinetics, benzene and chlorinated solvents would most likely cause liver cancer, lymphoma, or leukemia (Janeich *et al.* 1981). Although these contaminants were present in high concentrations at some locations, it was uncertain whether this resulted in significant exposure to Love Canal residents. A study of cancer rates at the site was conducted. Cancer incidence data were split into pre- and post-1966 census information because the quality of data from the New York Cancer Registry improved considerably in 1966. Data were then adjusted for age differences and tabulated separately for the sexes.

Table 3.1. Cancer incidence for residents of Love Canal as compared to expected incidences

	Males			Females		
Cancer	Observed	Expected	95% CI	Observed	Expected	95% CI
(A) 1955 to 1965						
Liver	0	0.4	0 to 2	2	0.3	0 to 1[1]
Lymphomas	3	2.5	0 to 5	2	1.8	0 to 4
Leukemias	2	2.3	0 to 5	3	1.7	0 to 4
(B) 1966 to 1977						
Liver	2	0.6	0 to 2	0	0.4	0 to 2
Lymphomas	0	3.2	0 to 6	4	2.5	0 to 5
Leukemias	1	2.5	0 to 5	2	1.8	0 to 4
(C) 1955 to 1977						
Liver	2	1.0	0 to 3	2	0.7	0 to 2
Lymphomas	3	5.6	2 to 11	6	4.3	1 to 8
Leukemias	3	4.8	1 to 9	5	3.5	0 to 7

[1] Although appearing significant, the linkage of the waste chemicals and liver cancer is unlikely as the two liver cancer victims lived in a Love Canal tract away from the waste location.

Table 3.1 provides documented cancer incidences for residents compared to expected incidences based on those for New York state (excluding New York City) for the same period (Janeich *et al.* 1981). Despite the perceived risks by residents and the Picciano report of elevated numbers of chromosomal aberrations, there were no obvious (statistically significant) increases in risk of these cancers associated with living at Love Canal (Figure 3.1). The perceived risk was inconsistent with the actual risk of cancer from the wastes. (Actual risk was estimated as the difference in expected and observed cancer incidence rates.) Nevertheless, considerable amounts of money were spent moving many families away from the area.

Cancer incidence rate ratio: nasal and lung cancer in nickel workers

A classic study of job-related nasal and lung cancer in Welsh nickel refinery workers will be used to illustrate the application of rate ratios in assessing disease in a human subpopulation. Doll, Morgan and Speizer (1970) documented

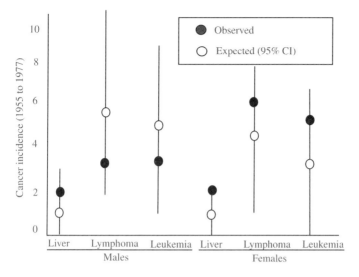

Fig. 3.1. Cancer incidence rates (1955 to 1977) associated with the Love Canal community (●) compared to those expected for New York State (exclusive of New York City) (○). Vertical lines around the expected rates are 95% confidence intervals

the cancer incidence ratio of nickel workers, and Welshmen and Englishmen of similar ages who were employed in other occupations. Data included information gathered after exposure control measures were instituted *circa* 1920–1925. Table 3.2. summarizes these data. Immediately obvious from the rate ratios is that nasal cancer deaths prior to 1925 were 116 to 870 times higher for nickel workers than for other men of similar age (Figure 3.2). After exposure controls were implemented, deaths from nasal cancer were not detected in the nickel

Table 3.2. Lung and nasal cancer in nickel industry workers versus men of England and Wales of other occupations. (Modified from Tables I and II of Doll, Morgan and Speizer 1970)

Year of first employment	Number of men	Number of person-years[1]	Nasal cancer cases Observed	Nasal cancer cases Expected	Ratio of rates	Lung cancer cases Observed	Lung cancer cases Expected	Ratio of rates
Before 1910	96	955.5	8	0.026	308	20	2.11	9.5
1910–1914	130	1060.5	20	0.023	870	29	2.75	10.5
1915–1919	87	915.0	6	0.015	400	13	2.29	5.7
1920–1924	250	1923.0	5	0.043	116	43	6.79	6.3
1925–1929	77	1136.0	0	0.014	—[2]	4	2.27	1.8
1930–1944	205	2945.0	0	0.022	—[2]	4	3.79	1.1

[1]Number of person-years at risk (1939–1966).
[2]Ratio of rate cannot be calculated because observed rate is 0.

workers. Similarly, lung cancer deaths were much higher in nickel workers before installation of control measures but dropped to levels similar to men in other occupations after exposure control. The risk ratios clearly demonstrated a heightened risk to nickel-processing workers and a tremendous drop in this risk after exposure control measures were established.

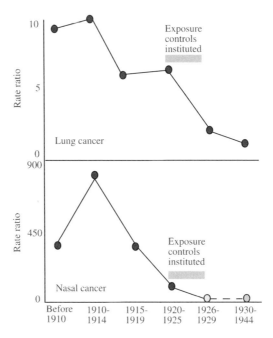

Fig. 3.2. Rate ratios for lung and nasal cancers in nickel workers compared to English and Welsh workers in other occupations. The rate ratios for both cancers dropped for nickel workers as measures to reduce exposure via particulates were instituted beginning in approximately 1920

Relative risk can be expressed as an odds ratio (OR) in case–control studies. Case–control studies identify individuals with the disease and then establish an appropriate control group. The status of individuals in each group relative to some risk factor, e.g. exposure to a chemical, is then established and possible linkage assessed between the risk factor and disease.

Odds are simply the probability of having (p) the disease divided by the probability of not having ($1 - p$) the disease, i.e. $p/(1 - p)$. The number of disease cases (individuals) that were (a) or were not (b) exposed, and the number of control individuals free of the disease that were (c) or were not (d) exposed to the risk factor are used to estimate the odds ratio (Ahlbom 1993; Sahai and Khurshid 1996):

$$\text{Odds ratio} = \frac{a/b}{c/d} = \frac{ad}{bc} \qquad (3.10)$$

For illustration, let's assume that a disease was documented in 50 individuals: 40 cases were associated with individuals previously exposed to a toxicant (a) and 10 of them (b) were associated with people never exposed to the chemical. In a control or reference sample of 75 people with no signs of the disease, 20 had been exposed (c) and 55 (d) had no known exposure. The odds ratio in this study would be (40)(55)/(10)(20) or 11. This odds ratio suggests that exposure to this chemical influences proneness to the disease: an individual's odds of getting the disease was eleven times higher if they had been exposed to the chemical.

Approximate variance and confidence intervals for the odds ratio can be generated from those for the natural logarithm of the odds ratio (Ahlbom 1993; Sahai and Khurshid 1996):

$$\ln \text{ OR} = \ln \frac{a}{N_1 - a} - \ln \frac{c}{N_0 - c} \tag{3.11}$$

where N_1 and N_0 are the number of cases (individuals) in the exposed and control groups, respectively:

$$\text{Variance of } \ln \text{ OR} \approx \frac{1}{a} + \frac{1}{b} + \frac{1}{c} + \frac{1}{d} \tag{3.12}$$

The confidence limits for ln OR can be approximated with

$$\ln \text{of OR} \pm Z_{\alpha/2} \sqrt{\frac{1}{a} + \frac{1}{b} + \frac{1}{c} + \frac{1}{d}} \tag{3.13}$$

As useful as these tools are for analyzing observational data, it is necessary to keep in mind the inherently compromised capacity to infer causal association with the context from which the observations are derived. Although the difficulties in inferring causation from observational data may be obvious, we will continue to emphasize them as epidemiological studies may be particularly vulnerable to this flaw. As an example of the caution required in applying observational information to inferring linkage between a potential risk factor and disease, Taubes (1995) provides a thorough explanation of the difficulties of taking any action, including communicating risk to the public, based on such studies. He describes several cancer risk factors arising from valid and highly publicized, but inferentially weak, studies (Table 3.3).

3.1.3 FOUNDATION MODELS DESCRIBING DISEASE IN POPULATIONS

Numerous models exist for describing disease in populations and potential relationships with etiological agents such as toxicants. Easily accessible textbooks such as those written by Ahlbom (1993), Marubini and Valsecchi (1995) and Sahai and Khurshid (1996) describe statistical models applicable to epidemiological data. Although most models focus on human epidemiology and clinical

Table 3.3. Examples of weak risk factors for human cancer

Risk factor	Relative risk	Cancer type
High-cholesterol diet	1.65	Rectal cancer in men
Eating yogurt more than once/month	2	Ovarian cancer
Smoking more than 100 cigarettes/lifetime	1.2	Breast cancer
High-fat diet	2	Breast cancer
Regular use of high-alcohol mouthwash	1.5	Mouth cancer
Vasectomy	1.6	Prostate cancer
Drinking >3.3 liters of (chlorinated?) fluid/day	2–4	Bladder cancer
Psychological stress at work	5.5	Colorectal cancer
Eating red meat five or more times/week	2.5	Colon cancer
On-job exposure to electromagnetic fields	1.38	Breast cancer
Smoking two packs of cigarettes daily	1.74	Fatal breast cancer

studies, there are no inherent obstacles to their wider application in ecological epidemiology. Regardless, most remain underutilized in ecotoxicology. The most important are described below.

3.1.3.1 Accelerated Failure Time and Proportional Hazard Models

Accelerated failure time and proportional hazard models are used to estimate the magnitude of effects, test for the statistical significance of risk factors including contaminant exposure concentration, and express these effects as probabilities or relative risks. This is done by modeling discrete events that occur through time such as time-to-death, time-to-develop cancer, time-to-disease onset, or time-to-symptom presentation (Figure 3.3).

The terms survival, mortality, and hazard functions need explanation before specific methods can be described. Let's begin our description of these terms and concepts by assuming an exposure time course with individuals dying during a period, T. The mortality of individuals within the population or cohort can be expressed by a probability density function ($f(t)$) and cumulative distribution function ($F(t)$). The straightforward estimate of the cumulative mortality or $F(t)$ is the total number of individuals dead at time, t, divided by the total number of exposed individuals:

$$\hat{F}(t) = \frac{\text{Number dead}_t}{\text{Total number exposed}} \tag{3.14}$$

Equally intuitive, the cumulative survival function ($S(t)$) is the number of individuals surviving to t divided by the total number of individuals exposed to the toxicant or, expressed in terms of $F(t)$,

$$\hat{S}(t) = 1 - F(t) \tag{3.15}$$

The hazard rate or function ($h(t)$) is the rate of deaths occurring during a time interval for all individuals that had survived to the beginning of that interval.

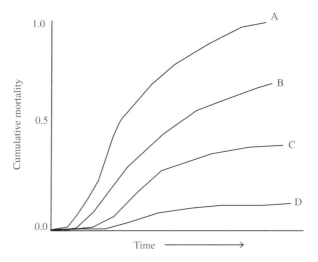

Fig. 3.3. Data resulting from a time-to-event analysis. Several treatments (A to D) are studied relative to time-to-death. Cumulative mortality of individuals in each treatment is plotted against duration of exposure (time)

The hazard rate has also been called the force of mortality, instantaneous failure or mortality rate, or proneness to fail. It is definable in terms of $f(t)$ and $F(t)$, or $S(t)$:

$$\hat{h}(t) = \frac{f(t)}{1 - F(t)} = \frac{-1}{S(t)} \frac{\mathrm{d}S(t)}{\mathrm{d}t} \tag{3.16}$$

The cumulative hazard function, $H(t)$, can be estimated from cumulative mortality $(F(t))$:

$$H(t) = \int_{-\infty}^{t} h(t)\mathrm{d}t = -\ln(1 - F(t)) \tag{3.17}$$

By simple rearrangement of equation (3.17) cumulative mortality can be expressed in terms of $H(t)$:

$$F(t) = 1 - \mathrm{e}^{-H(t)} \tag{3.18}$$

Note that, although death is being used in this description of terms, other events may be analyzed with these methods. Events may be any 'qualitative change that can be situated in time' (Allison 1995). The only restriction is that a discrete event occurs. Often the assumption is made that the event occurs only once, e.g. death. However, modifications to these methods allow accommodation for deviations from this condition, e.g. events such as giving birth that can occur more than once for an individual.

Life (actuarial) table and product-limit (Kaplan–Meier) methods are the two most commonly used nonparametric approaches for time-to-death analysis. Bootstrapping methods can also be applied (Manly in press) but will not be discussed. None of these methods requires a specific form for the underlying survival distribution. Actuarial tables produce estimates of $S(t)$ for a fixed sequence of intervals, e.g. yearly age classes of humans. Miller (1981) provides a basic discussion of computations for applying life tables in epidemiology. Life tables are discussed in more detail in Chapter 5. With the product-limit approach, the time intervals can vary in length. General details for this method are given below with additional information available from Miller (1981), Cox and Oakes (1984), and Marubini and Valsecchi (1995).

The product-limit estimate of $S(t)$ was originally described by Kaplan and Meier (1958) and an associated maximum likelihood method by Kalbfleisch and Prentice (1980). The notation here is that applied in widely used manuals of the SAS Institute (SAS 1989):

$$\hat{S}(t_i) = \prod_{j=1}^{i} \left(1 - \frac{d_j}{n_j} \right) \tag{3.19}$$

where $i =$ indicates that there are i failure times, t_i,

$n_j =$ the number of individuals alive just before t_j, and

$d_j =$ the number of individuals dying at time, t_j.

Although this product-limit estimate of $S(t)$ is appropriate for all times up to the end of the exposure (T), it must remain undefined for times after T if there were survivors. (The Π function in equation (3.19) is similar to the Σ function except the product is taken over the i observations instead of the sum.)

The variance for the product-limit estimate is generated using Greenwood's formula

$$\hat{\sigma}^2 = \hat{S}(t_i)^2 \sum_{j=1}^{i} \frac{d_i}{n_j s_j} \tag{3.20}$$

where $s_j = n_j - d_j$. (Note that this equation is incorrect in Newman (1995) and Newman and Dixon (1996) because $\hat{S}(t_i)^2$ was unintentionally omitted from the formula.) Greenwood's estimate of variance reduces to equation (3.21) for all times before T if there was no censoring before termination of the experiment, i.e. survival times are known for all individuals dying before T (Dixon and Newman 1991):

$$\hat{\sigma}(t_j) = \frac{\hat{S}(t_j)[1 - \hat{S}(t_j)]}{N} \tag{3.21}$$

where $N =$ the total number of individuals exposed.

The confidence interval for these estimates can be generated using the square root of the variance estimated in equations (3.20) or (3.21) in

$$CI = \hat{S}(t_j) \pm z_{\alpha/2}\hat{\sigma}_j \tag{3.22}$$

These methods allow estimation of $S(t)$ for a group of individuals. Resulting survival curves for different classes (e.g. toxicant exposed versus unexposed) can be tested for equivalence with nonparametric methods. The log-rank and Wilcoxon rank tests check for evidence that the observed times-to-death for the various classes did not come from the same distribution.

Time-to-event data can also be analyzed with semi-parametric and parametric methods. These semi-parametric and fully parametric models are expressed either as proportional hazard or accelerated failure time models. With proportional hazard models, the hazard of a reference group or type is used as a baseline hazard and the hazard of another group is scaled (made proportional) to that baseline hazard. For example, the hazard of contracting a liver cancer for fish living in a creosote-contaminated site might be made proportional to the baseline hazard for fish living in an uncontaminated site. A statement might be made that the hazard is ten times higher than that of the reference population. The hazards remain proportional by the same amount among classes regardless of the duration of exposure. In contrast, accelerated failure models use functions that describe the change in ln time-to-death resulting from some change in covariates. As with porportional hazard models, covariates can be class variables such as site or continuous variables such as animal weight. Hazards do not necessarily remain proportional by the same amount through time with accelerated failure time models. Continuing the example, the effect of creosote contamination on ln time-to-fatal cancer might be estimated with an accelerated failure model. The median time-to-fatal cancer appearance might be 230 days earlier than that of the reference population. Both forms of survival models are described below.

The general expression of a proportional hazard model is the following:

$$h(t, x_i) = e^{f(x_i)}h_0(t) \tag{3.23}$$

where $h(t, x_i) =$ the hazard at time t for a group or individual characterized with value x_i for the covariate x

$h_0(t) =$ the baseline hazard and

$e^{f(x_i)} =$ some function relating $h(t, x_i)$ to the baseline hazard.

The $f(x_i)$ is some function used to fit a continuous variable such as animal weight or a class variable such as exposure status. A vector of coefficients and a matrix of covariates can be included if more than one covariate is required.

The proportional hazard models described above assume that a specific distribution fits the baseline hazard $(h_0(t))$ and that hazards among classes remain proportional regardless of time (t). But a specified distribution for the baseline hazard is not an essential feature of proportional hazard models. A semi-parametric Cox proportional hazard model can be applied if the distribution was not apparent or was irrelevant to the needs of the study. This model retains the assumption of proportional hazard but empirically fits a (Lehmann) set of functions to the baseline hazard. No specific model is needed to describe the baseline hazard. Cox proportional hazard models are commonly applied in epidemiology because, in many cases, the underlying distribution is unimportant and the relative hazards for the classes are more important to understand.

As already mentioned, another form of survival model is the accelerated failure time model. In this case, the ln time-to-death is modified by $f(x_i)$:

$$\ln t_i = f(x_i) + \varepsilon_i \qquad (3.24)$$

where t_i = the time-to-death

$f(x_i)$ = a function that relates $\ln t_i$ to the covariate(s) and

ε_i = the error term.

3.1.3.2 Binary Logistic Regression Model

Logistic regression of a binary response variable (e.g. disease present or not, or individual dead or alive) can be used for analyzing epidemiological data associated with contamination. It is one of the most common approaches for analyzing epidemiological data of human disease (SAS 1995). The resulting statistical model predicts the probability of a disease occurrence based on values for risk factors:

$$\text{Prob } (Y = 1|X) = [1 + e^{-XB}]^{-1} \qquad (3.25)$$

The probability of a disease, e.g. a cancer ($Y = 1$), given a vector of risk factors (X) is predicted with the logistic function ($P = [1 + e^{-xB}]^{-1}$) where XB is $B_0 + B_1X_1 + B_2X_2 + B_3X_3 + \cdots B_kX_k$. The B values are the regression coefficients for the effects of the potential risk factors or etiological agents (X values).

One can also express the logistic model directly in terms of the logarithm of the odds ratio (Ahlbom 1993). In the equation below, the $\ln (P/(1 - P))$ transformation is the logit or ln of the odds of the disease occurring:

$$\ln \frac{P}{1 - P} = \alpha + XB \qquad (3.26)$$

Like results of the time-to-event models, the results of the logistic regression allow informed judgements about (1) potential agents that contribute to disease occurrence, (2) the probability of disease occurring given the presence of some agent or risk factor, and (3) the contribution of the agent or risk factor to the chance of disease occurrence relative to those of other agents or risk factors.

3.2 DISEASE ASSOCIATION AND CAUSATION

3.2.1 HILL'S NINE ASPECTS OF DISEASE ASSOCIATION

Emerging from the logic of causation (Section 3.1.1) are specific rules for enhancing belief in the association of noninfectious disease with chemical exposure. Sir Austin Hill (1965) provides one of the clearest and most relevant set of rules. They are meant to be used together to enhance belief but they are not rigid hypotheses that, if rejected, lead to only one conclusion. Hill's nine aspects of disease association are the following:

• A strong association enhances belief.

• Consistency of an observed association enhances belief.

• Specificity of an association can enhance belief.

• Consistent temporal sequence (cause present as a precondition to seeing the disease or high incidence of the disease) can enhance belief.

• A biological gradient (higher amounts produce higher levels or chance of effect) can enhance belief.

• Existence of a plausible biological mechanism can enhance belief.

• Coherence with our general knowledge base can enhance belief.

• Presence of experimental evidence can greatly enhance belief.

• Analogy drawn from another disease-causing agent can enhance belief.

Strength of association is very important in Hill's opinion. For instance, belief in association between smoking and lung cancer is greatly increased if one sees an incidence of lung cancer-related deaths that is 30 times higher for heavy smokers than nonsmokers. Similarly, the very high incidence of imposex (imposition of male characters like a penis and vas deferens on female individuals) in populations of the snail, *Nucella lapillus* from regions of coastal England with high concentrations of the antifouling agent, tributyltin (TBT) greatly reinforces belief that TBT causes imposex (Bryan and Gibbs 1991). However, it alone does not prove TBT is the causative agent.

Consistency of the association is also very important. Is there a higher incidence of lung cancer-related deaths in smokers versus nonsmokers regardless of ethnicity, sex, or cigarette brand? Here and elsewhere in this approach, it is important to be mindful of possible correlations with other factors. For example, in a study of correlations between smoking and cardiovascular disease, it would be useful to know if smokers tend to exercise less than nonsmokers. Lack of exercise, not smoking *per se*, could be the reason for increased cardiovascular disease in smokers. For the TBT-imposex example, documentation of imposex in more than 40 species of neogastropods from TBT-contaminated locations around the world (Bryan and Gibbs 1991; Poloczanka and Ansell 1999) reinforces belief that TBT causes imposex in *Nucella lapillus* populations. Tributyltin was a major component of marine paints used on boat and ship hulls. Therefore, TBT concentrations rise with increasing levels of boating and shipping activities in harbors, estuaries and bays. Certainly, other possible etiological agents also increase with increasing boating and shipping traffic activities. However, TBT is also used in plastics production and belief would be fostered by the presence of imposex in neogastropod populations inhabiting aquatic systems influenced by the plastics industry.

Belief is fostered if the disease emerges from very specific conditions, e.g. a specific toxicant is present in the air of a particular working environment in which a disease is seen in high incidence. A good example of disease emergence from specific conditions might be the extreme susceptibility of raptors and piscivorous birds to effects of DDT, a chemical with a high capacity to biomagnify through trophic levels (Woodwell 1967). Reproductive failure of top avian predators, but not birds lower in the trophic web, reinforced belief that a high concentration of DDT due to biomagnification was the cause of avian reproductive damage.

Temporal sequence is obviously important. It is logically mandatory that an effect not appear before the cause is present (Last 1983). But the exact time of exposure is difficult to define in some contaminant-induced diseases. Exposure over a long period may be required before a disease is manifest: there may be a long latency period between exposure to a carcinogen and the appearance of cancer. Regardless, temporal succession is central to causation as discussed above and is extremely helpful if obvious. Continuing the DDT example, belief was greatly enhanced by the close correspondence between the rapid decline in certain bird populations throughout the world and the onset of widespread use of DDT. Further, the recovery of certain bird populations such as osprey (*Pandion haliaetus*) (Spitzer *et al.* 1978) corresponded closely with the general ban on DDT use.

A clear biological gradient, such as an increased concentration of a toxicant correlated with an increase in effect, fosters belief, although it may not be necessary in order to assign an association between an etiological agent and a disease. For example, the observation that prevalence of *Nucella lapillus* imposex increases with proximity to TBT-contaminated harbors (Bryan and Gibbs 1991) reinforces the suggestion that TBT is the cause of imposex in this neogastropod. Other biological gradients can be more difficult to document. Some concentration–effect relationships have threshold concentrations below which there may be no discernable effect. Also, accurate measurement or estimation of exposure concentration can be extremely difficult and preclude establishment of a biological gradient.

Existence of a plausible biological mechanism can enhance belief as already discussed in our exploration of microexplanation (Chapter 1). The discovery that DDT and DDE interfered with ATPase enzymes critical to calcium deposition in the shell gland and resulted in excessively fragile eggs greatly enhanced our belief that DDT was the cause of reproductive failure in populations of birds (Simkiss

1996). As discussed in Chapter 2, the mechanism of differential bird predation on color morphs of peppered moths greatly fostered belief in the phenomenon of industrial melanism.

Biological plausibility is not always essential at initial phases of enhancing belief in disease association with some noninfectious agents. Limited knowledge may preclude ready assignment of biological plausibility in some cases.

Coherence with known facts is important regardless of our ability to identify a plausible mechanism. Baker *et al.* (1996) studied genetic damage to voles living around the Chernobyl reactor. They found extraordinary base-pair substitution rates for the mitochondrial cytochrome b gene: rates were orders-of-magnitude higher than expected. This very high mutation rate and the apparent viability of the vole populations seemed inconsistent with prevailing knowledge of mutation and cancer rates associated with radiation (see Hinton 1998 for details). High substitution rates in other genes are often associated with dysfunction. In fact, Baker *et al.* (1997) retracted their findings after realizing that an error had been made while reading associated DNA sequences. Belief was correctly hindered by a lack of coherence with existing biological knowledge. It caused the authors to go back and more carefully review their data.

Experimental results, as we have noted, have high inferential strength if produced and interpreted competently. Such results can be very useful in assigning association or enhancing belief. Experimental information is rare or its generation is often unethical in human epidemiology. In those instances in which some 'natural experiment' has occurred, the associated information can be applied in a very powerful way. This is much less of an obstacle in ecotoxicology because experimental data supporting the accumulation of knowledge about disease association is much more abundant.

Analogy can increase confidence in an association. Our present knowledge of the developmental effects of thalidomide to humans makes us more likely to believe in the potential effects of other chemicals on embryonic development. The early discovery of DDT biomagnification to harmful levels allowed more rapid acceptance of similar biomagnification and effects of other contaminants such as polychlorinated biphenyls (Evans, Noguchi and Rice 1991), toxophene (Evans, Noguchi and Rice 1991), and dibenzo-p-dioxins and -dibenzofurans (Broman *et al.* 1992; Rolff *et al.* 1993):

Here then are nine different viewpoints from all of which we should study association before we cry causation. What I do not believe — and this has been suggested — is that we can usefully lay down some hard-and-fast rules of evidence that must be obeyed before we accept cause and effect. None of my nine viewpoints can bring indisputable evidence for or against the cause-and-effect hypothesis and none are required as sine qua non. What they do, with greater or less strength, is to help us to make up our minds on the fundamental question — is there any other way of explaining the set of facts before us, is there any other answer equally, or more, likely than cause and effect? (Hill 1965)

Hill's nine aspects of disease association are simply specific points consistent with the general characteristics of causation. Other sets of rules exist in addition to Hill's, including Evans's postulates (Evans 1976) which are relevant extensions of Koch's postulates. Both Hill and Evans attempt to compensate a bit for the high dimensionality and less structured experimental context which slows 'the movement of thought toward belief' (Josephson and Josephson 1996). Regardless, only a subjective measurement is available for expression of confidence in the final assessment.

Box 3.2 Hockey sticks, mud, and fish livers: Hill's nine aspects of disease association

Let's illustrate the application of Hill's nine aspects of disease association with information gathered for hepatic cancer prevalence in English sole (*Pleuronectes vetulus*) populations of Puget Sound (Washington). During the 1970s, surveys began of bottom-dwelling fish in bays, estuaries and inlets of Puget Sound. Biological qualities (tissue lesions, demographic qualities, and biomarkers of effect and exposure) and chemical qualities (sediment and fish tissue PAH and other pollutant concentrations, and fluorescent aromatic compounds in bile) were measured at a series of contaminated and clean sites (Myers *et al.* 1990). Some supportive laboratory experiments were also conducted. This information was compared to the published literature, primarily the mammalian literature and is evaluated here according to Hill's nine aspects.

(1) *Strength of association enhances belief*: Horness *et al.* (1998) analyzed data for English sole inhabiting areas with sediment concentrations of polycyclic aromatic hydrocarbons ranging from 0 to 6300 ng/g dry weight of sediment. At the lowest concentrations, the prevalence of all types of liver lesions was extremely low but increased to approximately 60% at the most contaminated sites. Similarly, prevalence of neoplastic lesions was very high (*circa* 10%) at the most contaminated sites relative to the clean sites.

(2) *Consistency of an observed association enhances belief*: A consistent increase in lesion prevalence in English sole is seen at contaminated sites (Myers *et al.* 1990, 1994; Horness *et al.* 1998). This statement is valid for various lesion types reflecting a progression toward hepatic neoplasia including necrotic ⟶ proliferative ⟶ preneoplastic ⟶ neoplastic lesions. Necrotic lesions were thought to reflect cytotoxic effects of polycyclic aromatic hydrocarbons and their metabolites. Proliferative lesions reflect cell proliferation in compensation for this cytotoxicity. Neoplasia can eventually arise from the cells involved in this proliferation. Preneoplastic ('foci of cellular alteration') and neoplastic

lesions eventually appear as altered cells increase in numbers and tumors become apparent in the liver. Close examination of lesions by transmission electron microscopy revealed no evidence of viral infection (Myers *et al.* 1990), i.e. the cancers did not seem to be caused by a viral agent.

(3) *Specificity of an association can enhance belief*: Using logistic regression, hepatic lesion prevalences in English sole from a series of Pacific Coast sites were compared to a variety of contaminants in sediments (i.e. low molecular weight polycyclic aromatic hydrocarbons, high molecular weight polycyclic aromatic hydrocarbons, polychlorinated biphenyls, DDT and its derivatives, chlordanes, dieldrin, hexachlorobenzene, and several metals) (Myer *et al.* 1994). The polycyclic aromatic hydrocarbons, polychlorinated biphenyls, DDT and its derivatives, chlordane and dieldrin were all found to be significant risk factors. This suggests that specificity may not be high for this association.

(4) *Consistent temporal sequence can enhance belief*: The field studies could not address this aspect directly. This reflects the common challenge with chemical carcinogenesis because the ability to make a temporal linkage is hampered by the characteristically long period of cancer latency. Regardless, an appropriate temporal sequence was suggested by the observation that neoplastic lesions were not often seen in field-collected young sole but lesions thought to occur early in the progression toward neoplasia were found in these young sole (Myers *et al.* 1990, 1998). Laboratory experiments suggested that the exposure to polycyclic aromatic hydrocarbons resulted in lesions characteristic of early stages of a progression toward liver neoplasia (Myers *et al.* 1990).

(5) *A biological gradient can enhance belief*: Figure 3.4 shows the consistent threshold ('hockey-stick') exposure–effect curve for polycyclic aromatic hydrocarbons versus preneoplastic ('foci of cellular alteration') and neoplastic lesions in sole liver. A biological gradient with a threshold is suggested in the reports of Myers *et al.* (1998) and Horness *et al.* (1998).

(6) *Existence of a plausible biological mechanism can enhance belief*: A clear mechanism for liver neoplasia appearance exists based on P450-mediated production of free radicals which form DNA adducts. Such adduct formation was clearly documented in English sole from contaminated sites and was correlated with lesions thought to lead to neoplasia (Myers *et al.* 1998).

(7) *Coherence with general knowledge can enhance belief*: The results described for English sole are consistent with a wide literature concerning chemical carcinogenesis including specifics of polycyclic aromatic hydrocarbon induction of cancers in diverse animal models (Moore and Myers

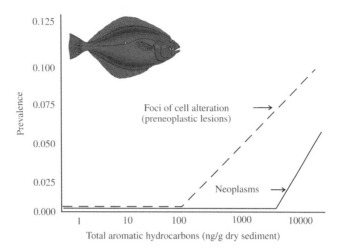

Fig. 3.4. Prevalence of foci of cellular alteration (preneoplastic lesions) and neoplastic lesions in livers of English sole (*Pleuronectes vetulus*) sampled from areas with widely differing sediment concentrations of aromatic hydrocarbons. Note the clear threshold or 'hockey stick' dose–response curve for both types of lesions. (This figure combines information from Figures 1A and B of Horness *et al.* 1998)

1994). The lesion progression described for English sole closely parallels that described for rodents (Myers *et al.* 1990).

(8) *Presence of experimental evidence can greatly enhance belief*: As mentioned above, laboratory exposure to polycyclic aromatic hydrocarbons resulted in lesions indicative of a progression toward hepatic neoplasia (Myers *et al.* 1998).

(9) *Analogy drawn from another disease-causing agent can enhance belief*: The specific findings regarding hepatic tumor appearance in English sole following exposure to polycyclic aromatic hydrocarbons are consistent with a diverse literature on chemical carcinogenesis.

In summary, the information available for hepatic cancer in English sole from the Puget Sound area strongly supports its association with polycyclic aromatic hydrocarbon contamination. The only aspects that do not strongly support this association are the nonspecificity of hepatic cancer and the lack of a clearly documented temporal sequence because the time required between exposure and full expression of a neoplastic lesion is so long. However, laboratory studies with sole show a progression after exposure to lesions leading to cancer, and studies with other fishes more amenable to laboratory manipulation have documented a consistent temporal sequence from polycyclic aromatic hydrocarbon exposure and liver cancer (Moore and Myers

1994). It would be very difficult to state that the other carcinogens noted above were not contributing risk factors also. Regardless, the preponderance of evidence suggests that polycyclic aromatic hydrocarbons play a dominant role in determining the prevalence of hepatic cancer in English sole.

Clearly, some methods are better than others for extracting epidemiological information from populations. Also some exploration methods are better than others for gathering evidence of disease association in populations. The strength of evidence hierarchy described below focuses on the inferential value of evidence emerging from different types of studies.

3.2.2 STRENGTH OF EVIDENCE HIERARCHY

All epidemiological evidence is not equally valuable for determining the true state of a cause–effect relationship. As we have already discussed, causal relationships are often defined as much by context as objective reality. For instance, factors leading to human disease can be categorized based on context (Last 1983) as either predisposing, enabling, precipitating, or reinforcing factors. Predisposing factors create a situation conducive to disease appearance. For example, a chemical that causes immune suppression could be envisioned as a predisposing factor for the development of infectious disease. Enabling factors are those fostering or diminishing the expression of disease. They contribute by making the individual more or less inclined to be in some state that positively or negatively influences the chance of disease. For example, poverty-related, poor nutrition may allow disease to be manifested or, conversely, high income-related use of health services may be correlated with more rapid recovery from disease. Economic status may be an enabling factor for some human diseases. Precipitating factors are those associated with the clear onset of disease such as high exposure to a toxicant in the work environment. Precipitating factors are often identified as 'causes' of disease. Reinforcing factors tend to encourage the appearance of or prolong the duration of disease. Creation of a marginal habitat with multiple 'stressors' during remediation in addition to a residual level of toxicant may reinforce the manifestation of disease in a population. Frequent foraging of a species in a contaminated environment may also be a reinforcing factor for disease.

Upon careful review of the characteristics of causation, it is clear that these overlapping distinctions are based partially on experimental context and partially on how closely a factor conforms to the qualities of a causative agent. For example, a precipitating factor associated with disease is easily identified as the cause if it were necessary — must be present — for the disease to occur. (In the context of disease causation, the terms necessary and sufficient are given specific meanings. If something is necessary, it must always be present for the disease to be manifested. If something is sufficient, it will initiate or produce the disease. Its presence is sufficient for the disease to be expressed (Last 1983).) However, other factors may be equally necessary for the expression of disease and context could determine which of several necessary, precipitating factors caused the disease. At the other end of the spectrum, an enabling factor would be difficult to identify as the cause because disease can occur in its absence or may not occur in its presence. It is neither necessary nor sufficient.

Strength of evidence can be categorized based on the approach used to produce it (Green and Byar 1984). The weakest information emerges from anecdotal reports of disease. For example, contaminants were implicated in a die-off of seals (Dickson 1988). Dickson bolstered this implication by quoting Lies Vedder, a Dutch veterinary surgeon:

> *We have never seen so many problems with bacterial infections with seal pups as this year; for example, I have not seen a single healthy umbilical scar. There seems to be no way of treating them, and the immune system does not seem able to cope; we have no proof that there is immune suppression, but there are certainly signs.*

Although the implications could very easily be correct, this is fairly weak evidence for assigning causation. Better evidence is produced from case series without controls and even better evidence from case series with literature controls. The next best evidence comes from computer analyses of disease cases with consideration of disease expectations for unexposed individuals. Quality of evidence improves dramatically with the four approaches described next because they include formal control or reference cases. Case–control observational studies have already been discussed relative to odds ratios, e.g. equation (3.10). In such studies, information is collected for disease cases and appropriate controls ('references' or 'noncases') in the population for a specified interval. Even stronger inferences are derived from a series of studies based on historical control groups. Finally, more powerful evidence can be produced in clinical or experimental trials. These highly structured experiments are superior to any discussed to this point because of the ability to randomly assign observations to treatments and to control confounding factors. Opportunity for generation of this type of information is higher for nonhuman species than human species. A single, controlled laboratory study produces more powerful information than methods discussed above and the associated information is only inferior to that emerging from a series of confirming, controlled, and randomized laboratory studies. Again, careful examination will show that this hierarchy of strength of evidence emerges directly from the guidelines for determining the strength of inferences about cause-effect relationships (Section 3.1.1).

3.3 INFECTIOUS DISEASE AND TOXICANT-EXPOSED POPULATIONS

Odum (1971) described the principle of instant pathogen in which a sudden outbreak of disease is induced by either an introduction of rapidly reproducing species into a system lacking the ability to counterbalance its progress or a rapid change of the environment which tips the balance to favor the pathogen. Later, Odum (1985) listed a series of ecosystem alterations anticipated with chemical stress, including an increase in 'negative interactions', i.e. parasitism and disease. This theme of increased infectious disease with increased stress or pollution is repeated many times throughout the ecotoxicology literature.

The paradigm of the infectious disease triad provides an even more inclusive view of the influence of pollution on changes in infectious disease. As Figure 3.5 suggests, any environmental change can influence the outcome of the disease process. The final balance between health and disease is a result of environmental influences on both partners (host and infectious agent) in the disease process. As an example, summer oyster (*Crassostrea virginica*) mortality in Delaware Bay due to the sporozoan parasite, *Haplosporidium nelsoni*, depends on temperatures experienced during the preceding winter (Ford and Haskin 1982).

The triad paradigm for disease extends to environmental factors such as anthropogenic agents. Tributyltin oxide decreased oyster (*C. virginica*) resistance to the protozoan, *Perkinus marinus* (Fisher *et al.* 1999). Copper decreased catfish (*Ictalurus punctatus*) resistance to the protozoan, *Ichthyophthirius multifiliis* (Ewing, Ewing and Zimmer 1982). Extending the example of temperature's effects on disease outcome to the extreme case of thermal pollution, alligators (*Alligator mississippiensis*) inhabiting thermal effluents from nuclear reactors had diminished resistance to infection by the bacterium, *Aeromonas*

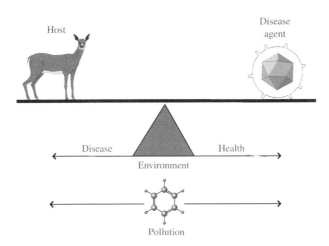

Fig. 3.5. The infectious disease triad paradigm in which environmental factors (the fulcrum here) can shift the balance of health-disease processes to favor the host or infectious agent. Pollutants, as components of the environment can also shift the fulcrum to favor the host or infectious agent. Together, natural and anthropogenic components in the environment determine the final balance in the health–disease process

hydrophilia (Glassman and Bennett 1978). Obviously, chemicals or physical agents compromising immunological competence such as some pesticides (Grant and Merhle 1973; Bennett and Wolke 1987) will influence the disease process (Anderson 1990).

Although the focus in the above discussion was the increase in likelihood of disease due to pollution, the infectious disease triad paradigm implies that changes in the environment can also tip the balance in favor of the host. For example, although high concentrations of some metals increased bacterial infection in striped bass (*Morone saxatilis*) by *Flexibacter columnaris*, elevated levels of other metals decreased infection (MacFarlane, Bullock and McLaughlin 1986). Copper and zinc reduced the longevity and infectivity of cercariae of the trematode, *Echinoparypium recurvatum*, suggesting a potential impact on parasite transmission (Evans 1982a). These metals also reduced shedding of *Notocotylus attenuatus* cercariae from the snail host (*Lymnaea stagnalis*) (Evans 1982b). Mortality of trout (*Salmo gairdneri*) from *Aeromonas hydrophila* infection was lower in individuals injected with low doses of PCBs than in controls, perhaps due to their increased blood leucocrits (Snarski 1982). In contrast to immunosuppression by contaminants, the trout response to infection seems to be a case of heightened immunological competence due to PCB injection before disease challenge. In these same studies, pre-exposure to copper did not influence disease outcome.

To summarize, pollutants are components of the complex milieu in which hosts and infectious agents interact. As such, they can influence the infectious disease process to favor the host or disease agent. This conclusion is consistent with the infectious disease triad paradigm and is more inclusive than Odum's (1971) principle of the instant pathogen. Regardless, such environmental influence on infectious disease is invoked primarily in speculations about infectious disease outbreaks (e.g. Dickson 1988; Sarokin and Schulkin 1992). More extensive ecotoxicological research into contaminant influences on infectious disease is needed.

3.4 DIFFERENCES IN SENSITIVITY WITHIN AND AMONG POPULATIONS

Differences in risk from contaminants exist among individuals in a population. As we will discuss in Chapter 8, some of these differences are related to the genetic qualities of individuals. Others are associated with changes occurring in an individual's life cycle, e.g. younger or older individuals may be more sensitive to a particular contaminant. Still others are associated with interactions between genetic and environmental qualities (Chapter 8). These differences can influence population characteristics and fate as described in the next few chapters. Because populations often occupy heterogeneous landscapes, differences in risk to contaminants may also occur on a spatial scale. In such cases, keystone habitats may play a critical role in determining the nature and persistence of the population. Ignoring these differences in populations can result in poor prediction of contaminant effects. The goal of the next several chapters is to provide ample understanding so that predictions of population effects can be made in such situations. Many of the methods described in this chapter can be combined with this understanding to describe and predict population effects of contaminants.

3.5 SUMMARY

In this chapter we explored concepts and metrics applied in epidemiology, the science of disease in populations. A brief review of the topics discussed should reveal a tendency to focus on individuals within populations and to emphasize risk to individuals. In the next few chapters we will explore methods designed specifically to project qualities of populations.

Logical and mathematical constructs were described for teasing out causation or strong association from epidemiological data. Respectively, Hill's aspects of disease association and the strength of evidence hierarchy were examined as the best means to infer disease association and to judge the inferential strength of evidence from diverse types of studies. The disease triad paradigm was selected as the most inclusive for understanding the influence of pollutants on the manifestation and outcome of infectious disease. Finally, we briefly described the factors that make individuals within a population more or less prone to the effects of pollutants.

3.5.1 SUMMARY OF FOUNDATION CONCEPTS AND PARADIGMS

- The descriptive nature of much epidemiological information results in relatively weak inferences.

- Strength of inferences can be enhanced by logical rules such as Hill's nine aspects of disease association and the value of evidence supporting inferences judged by the strength of evidence hierarchy.

- Mechanistic knowledge is not required for inferences about disease association but its existence greatly enhances inferential strength.

- Disease prevalence and incidence are sound metrics of disease dynamics in populations. Differences in these metrics within and among populations are useful in describing disease in populations.

- Some dose–effect relationships have thresholds while others do not.

- Binary logistic, accelerated failure time, and proportional hazard models are adequate to describe many toxicant exposure–disease associations.

- The likelihood of disease is a function of the interaction among the host, the disease agent, and the environment. Pollutants, as part of the environmental milieu in which the host and disease agent interact, can modify the likelihood of disease.

• Toxicants can weaken individuals (e.g. immunosuppression), resulting in an increase in infectious disease in the population. However, enhanced immunological competence is also possible due to pollutant exposure, resulting in a decrease in infection.

• Toxicants can increase or decrease parasite load as a complex function of relative toxicant effects to the host, parasite, or another host population.

• Individuals differ genetically relative to their risk of an adverse effect after toxicant exposure.

• Nongenetic risk factors also vary among individuals, resulting in differences in risk upon exposure.

• Populations can differ in their responses to toxicant exposure due to the differences in nongenetic and genetic risk factors of individuals in each population.

• Population differences in risk factors can lead to a keystone habitat or 'keystone population' context of effect in a landscape with a nonrandom distribution of contamination.

• Individuals can vary in risk of disease at different stages of their lives.

• Correlations of factors with disease within and among populations can result in incorrect inferences about association or causation.

REFERENCES

Ahlbom A (1993). *Biostatistics for Epidemiologists*. CRC/Lewis Publishers, Boca Raton, FL.

Allison PD (1995). *Survival Analysis Using the SAS System: A Practical Guide*. SAS Institute, Inc.: Cary, NC.

Anderson DP (1990). Immunological indicators: effects of environmental stress on immune protection and disease outbreaks. *Amer Fish Soc Sympos* **8**: 38–50.

Baker RJ, Van den Bussche RA, Wright AJ, Wiggins LE, Hamilton MJ, Reat EP, Smith MH, Lomakin MD and Chesser RK (1996). High levels of genetic change in rodents of Chernobyl. *Nature* **380**: 707–708.

Baker RJ, Van den Bussche RA, Wright AJ, Wiggins LE, Hamilton MJ, Reat EP, Smith MH, Lomakin MD and Chesser RK (1997). High levels of genetic change in rodents of Chernobyl — retraction. *Nature* **390**: 100.

Bennet RO and Wolke RE (1987). The effect of sublethal endrin exposure on rainbow trout, *Salmo gairdneri* Richardson. I. Evaluation of serum cortisol concentrations and immune responsiveness. *J Fish Biol* **31**: 375–385.

Broman D, Näf C, Rolff C, Zebühr Y, Fry B and Hobbie J (1992). Using ratios of stable nitrogen to estimate bioaccumulation and flux of polychlorinated dibenzo-p-dioxins (PCDDs). and dibenzofurans (PCDFs) in two food chains from the Northern Baltic. *Environ Toxicol Chem* **11**: 331–345.

Bryan GW and Gibbs PE (1991). Impact of low concentrations of tributyltin (TBT) on marine organisms: a review. In *Metal Ecotoxicology. Concepts & Applications*, ed. by MC Newman and AW McIntosh, pp. 323–361, CRC/Lewis Press, Chelsea, MI.

Cox DR and Oakes D (1984). *Analysis of Survival Data*. Chapman & Hall, London.
Culliton BJ (1980). Continuing confusion over Love Canal. *Science* **209**: 1002–1003.
Dickson, D. (1988). Mystery disease strikes Europe's seals. *Science* **241**: 893–895.
Dixon PM and Newman MC (1991). Analyzing toxicity data using statistical models for time-to-death: an introduction. In *Metal Ecotoxicology. Concepts & Applications*, ed. by Mc Newman and AW McIntosh, pp. 207–242. CRC/Lewis Press, Chelsea, MI.
Doll R, Morgan LG and Speizer FE (1970). Cancers of the lung and nasal sinuses in nickel workers. *Br J Cancer* **24**: 624–632.
Evans AS (1976). Causation and disease: the Henle–Koch postulates revisited. *Yale J Biol Med* **49**: 175–195.
Evans MS, Noguchi GE and Rice CP (1991). The biomagnification of polychlorinated biphenyls, toxaphene, and DDT compounds in a Lake Michigan offshore food web. *Arch Environ Contam Toxicol* **20**: 87–93.
Evans NA (1982a). Effect of copper and zinc upon the survival and infectivity of *Echinoparyphium recurvatum* cercariae. *Parasitology* **85**: 295–303.
Evans NA (1982b). Effects of copper and zinc on the life cycle of *Notocotylus attenuatus* (Digenea: Notocotylidae). *Inter J Parasit* **12**: 363–369.
Ewing MS, Ewing SA and Zimmer MA (1982). Sublethal copper stress and susceptibility of channel catfish to experimental infections with *Ichthyophthirius multifiliis*. *Bull Environm Contam Toxicol* **28**: 676–681.
Fisher WS, Oliver LM, Walker WW, Manning CS and Lytle TF (1999). Decreased resistance of eastern oysters (*Crassostrea virginica*) to a protozoan pathogen (*Perkinsus marinus*) after sublethal exposure to tributyltin oxide. *Mar Environ Res* **47**: 185–201.
Ford SE and Haskin HH (1982). History and epizootiology of *Haplosporidium nelsoni* (MSX), an oyster pathogen in Delaware Bay, 1957–1980. *J Invert Pathol* **40**: 118–141.
Glassman AB and Bennett CE (1978). Responses of the alligator to infection and thermal stress. In *Energy and Environmental Stress in Aquatic Systems*, ed. by JH Thorp and JW gibbons, pp. 691–702, National Technical Information Service, Springfield, VA.
Grant BF and Mehrle PM (1973). Endrin toxicosis in rainbow trout (*Salmo gairdneri*). *J Fish Res Bd Can* **30**: 31–40.
Green SB and Byar DP (1984). Using observational data from registries to compare treatments: the fallacy of omnimetrics. *Statistics in Medicine* **3**: 361–370.
Harré R. (1972). *The Philosophies of Science. In Introductory Survey*. Oxford University Press, Oxford.
Hill AB (1965). The environment and disease: Association or causation? *Proc R Soc Med* **58**: 295–300.
Hinton TG (1998). Estimating human and ecological risks from exposure to radiation. In *Risk Assessment. Logic and Measurement*, ed. by MC Newman and CL Strojan, pp. 143–166, CRC/Ann Arbor Press, Chelsea, MI.
Horness BH, Lomax DP, Johnson LL, Myers MS, Pierce SM and Collier TK (1998). Sediment quality thresholds: estimates from hockey stick regression of liver lesion prevalence in English sole (*Pleuronectes vetulus*). *Environ Toxicol Chem* **17**: 872–882.
Janeich DT, Burnett WS, Feck G, Hoff M, Nasca P, Polednak AP, Greenwald P and Vianna N (1981). Cancer incidence in the Love Canal area. *Science* **212**: 1404–1407.
Josephson JR and Josephson SG (1996). *Abductive Inference. Computation, Philosophy, Technology*. Cambridge University Press, Cambridge.
Kalbfleisch JD and Prentice RL (1980). *The Statistical Analysis of Failure Time Data*. John Wiley, New York.
Kant I. (1934). *Critique of Pure Reason*. JM Dent: London.
Kaplan EL and Meier P (1958). Nonparametric estimation from incomplete observations. *J Am Statist Assoc* **53**: 457–481.
Last JM (1983). *A Dictionary of Epidemiology*. Oxford University Press, Oxford.

Lipfert FW (1985). Mortality and air pollution: is there a meaningful connection? *Environ Sci Technol* **19**: 764–770.

Manly BFJ (in press) Time-to-event analyses in ecology. In *Can Risk Assessment be Improved with Time-to-Event Models?* ed. by PF Chapman, M Crane, T Sparks, MC Newman and J Fenlon, SETAC Press, Pensacola, FL.

Marubini E and Valsecchi MG (1995). *Analyzing Survival Data from Clinical Trials and Observational Studies*. John Wiley, Chichester.

MacFarlane RD, Bullock GL and McLaughlin JJA (1986). Effects of five metals on susceptibility of striped bass to *Flexibacter columnaris*. *Trans Amer Fish Soc* **115**: 227–231.

Miller Jr RG (1981). *Survival Analysis*. John Wiley, Chichester.

Moore MJ and Myers MS (1994). Pathobiology of chemical-associated neoplasia in fish. In *Aquatic Toxicology. Molecular, Biochemical and Cellular Perspectives*, ed. by DC Malins and GK Ostrander, pp. 327–386. CRC/Lewis Publishers, Boca Raton, FL.

Myers MS, Johnson LL, Hom T, Collier TK, Stein JE and Varanasi U (1998). Toxicopathic hepatic lesions in subadult English sole (*Pleuronectes vetulus*) from Puget Sound, Washington, USA: relationships with other biomarkers of contaminant exposure. *Mar Environ Res* **45**: 47–67.

Myers MS, Landahl JT, Krahn MM, Johnson LL and McCain BB (1990). Overview of studies on liver carcinogenesis in English sole from Puget Sound; Evidence for a xenobiotic chemical etiology I: Pathology and epizootiology. *Sci Total Environ* **94**: 33–50.

Myers MS, Stehr C, Olson OP, Johnson LL, McCain BB, Chan S-L and Varanasi U (1994). Relationships between toxicopathic hepatic lesions and exposure to chemical contaminants in English sole (*Pleuronectes vetulus*), starry flounder (*Platichthys stellatus*), and white croaker (*Genyonemus lineatus*) from selected marine sites on the Pacific Coast, USA. *Environ Health Perspect* **102**: 200–215.

Newman MC (1995). *Quantitative Methods in Aquatic Ecotoxicology*. CRC/Lewis Press, Boca Raton, FL.

Newman MC and Dixon PM (1996). Ecologically meaningful estimates of lethal effect in individuals. In *Ecotoxicology. A Hierarchical Treatment*, ed. by MC Newman and CH Jagoe, pp. 225–253. CRC/Lewis Press, Boca Raton, FL.

Odum EP (1971). *Fundamentals of Ecology*. WB. Saunders Co., Philadelphia, PA:

Odum EP (1985). Trends expected in stressed ecosystems. *Bioscience* **35**: 419–422.

Piattelli-Palmarini M. (1994). *Inevitable Illusions*. John Wiley, New York.

Poloczanska ES and Ansell AD (1999). Imposex in the whelks *Buccinum undatum* and *Neptunea antiqua* from the west coast of Scotland. *Mar Environ Res* **47**: 203–212.

Popper KA (1959). *The Logic of Scientific Discovery*. Routledge, New York.

Popper KA (1965). *Conjectures and Refutations: The Growth of Scientific Knowledge*. Harper and Row, London.

Rench JD (1994). Environmental epidemiology. In *Basic Environmental Toxicology*, ed. by LG Cockerham and BS Shane, pp. 477–499. CRC/Lewis Press, Boca Raton, FL.

Rolff C, Broman D, Näf C and Zebühr Y. (1993). Potential biomagnification of PCDD/Fs — New possibilities for quantitative assessment using stable isotope trophic position. *Chemosphere* **27**: 461–468.

Sahai H and Khurshid A (1996). *Statistics in Epidemiology. Methods, Techniques and Application*. CRC Press, Boca Raton, FL.

Sarokin D and Schulkin J (1992). The role of pollution in large-scale population disturbances. Part 1: aquatic populations. *Environ Sci Technol* **26**: 1476–1484.

SAS Institute Inc. (1989). *SAS/STAT User's Guide, Version 6, Fourth Edition, Volume 2*. SAS Institute Inc., Cary, NC.

SAS Institute Inc. (1995). *Logistic Regression Examples Using the SAS System, Version 6, First Edition.* SAS Institute Inc., Cary, NC.

Simkiss K (1996). Ecotoxicants at the cell-membrane barrier. In *Ecotoxicology. A Hierarchical Treatment,* ed. by MC Newman and CH Jagoe, pp. 59–83. CRC/Lewis Press, Boca Raton, FL.

Smith RJ (1982a). Love Canal study attracts criticism. *Science* **217**: 714–715.

Smith RJ (1982b). The risks of living near Love Canal. *Science* **217**: 808–811.

Snarski VM (1982). The response of rainbow trout *Salmo gairdneri* to *Aeromonas hydrophila* after sublethal exposures to PCB and copper. *Environ Pollut Ser A* **28**: 219–232.

Spitzer PR, Risebrough RW, Walker II W, Hernandez R, Poole A, Puleston D and Nisbet ICT (1978). Productivity of ospreys in Connecticut–Long Island increase as DDE residues decline. *Science* **202**: 333–335.

Suter II GW (1993). *Ecological Risk Assessment.* CRC/Lewis Press, Boca Raton, FL.

Taubes G (1995). Epidemiology faces its limits. *Science* **269**: 164–169.

Tversky A and Kahneman D (1992). Advances in prospect theory: cumulative representation of uncertainty. *J Risk and Uncertainty* **5**: 297–323.

Woodwell GM (1967). Toxic substances and ecological cycles. *Sci Am* **216**: 24–31.

4 Toxicants and Simple Population Models

4.1 TOXICANT EFFECTS ON POPULATION SIZE AND DYNAMICS

4.1.1 THE POPULATION-BASED PARADIGM FOR ECOLOGICAL RISK

...the greatest scandal of philosophy is that, while around us the world of nature perishes...philosophers continue to talk, sometimes cleverly and sometimes not, about the question of whether this world exists. (Popper, 1972)

According to Kuhn's *The Structure of Scientific Revolutions*, every scientific discipline is built around a collection of conceptual and methodological paradigms that are 'revealed in its textbooks, lectures and laboratory exercises' (Kuhn 1962). These paradigms define what the discipline encompasses — and what it does not. During professional training, a scientist also learns the rules by which business within her discipline is to be conducted. She understands that there is a 'hard core' of irrefutable beliefs that are not to be questioned and a 'protective belt of auxiliary hypotheses' that are actively tested and enriched (Lakatos 1970). A population biologist might test the hypothesis that microevolution occurs at a different rate in stressed populations than in unstressed populations, but not the validity of evolution by natural selection. To venture outside the accepted borders of a discipline or to question a core paradigm is courting professional censure. Yet, when a core paradigm fails too obviously and another is available to take its place, significant shifts in a discipline occur. Oddly enough, a clearly inadequate paradigm will remain central in a discipline if a better one isn't available to replace it (Braithwaite 1983). Because scientists are human, the shift from one core paradigm to another is characterized by as much discomfort and bickering as excitement. Einstein's dismissal of Heisenberg's principle of uncertainty with the retort that 'God doesn't play dice with the universe' demonstrates that even the best of scientists becomes peevish when a new paradigm is proposed to replace an existing central one. In a similar quip cited by Howson and Urbach (1989), after a student asked Einstein what he would have done if his theory of general relativity failed a particularly crucial test, he answered, 'Then I would have to pity the dear Lord. The theory is still correct.'

Resistance to abandon a failing context is not a singular foible of scientists. In the psychology of problem solving, such theory tenacity is evident in the resistance to abandon a candidate solution after it has proven to be untenable (Loehle 1987). Similar resistance is present in investment psychology as the endowment effect, the irrational resistance to take money out of a failing investment (Piattelli-Palmarini 1994). Regardless of its universality, it is a psychological habit to keep in mind as old paradigms are questioned and new paradigms arise.

Although originating from illogical roots, the dogmatic tendency to cling to a paradigm does have a positive consequence (Popper 1972). Any group of scientists who tend to drop a central paradigm too quickly will experience many disappointments and false starts. A key character of any scientific discipline is a healthy, but not pathological, tenacity of central paradigms.

In writing this and several of the remaining chapters, I am caught between the risk of being censured for discussing topics out of balance with their perceived importance in ecotoxicology and the conviction that ecotoxicologist are dawdling in accepting a useful, new core paradigm for evaluating ecological risk. Much like the negligent philosophers described in the quote above, ecotoxicologists are enjoying the exploration of the innumerable details of their protective belt of auxiliary paradigms and hypotheses while real questions about ecological risk remain poorly addressed by a core, individual-based paradigm for ecotoxicology. We need to focus less on individual-based metrics and more on population-based metrics of effect. This cannot be adequately done by superficially modifying the present paradigm that existing individual-based metrics accurately predict population consequences. Instead of adding to the protective belt around this collapsing paradigm, we need to work more toward producing population-level metrics of effects. Until this new population-level paradigm is more fully developed and sufficient detail is added to it, ecotoxicologists will maintain a failing one by jerry-building collectively acceptable irrationalities, e.g. the 96 h LC50 measure of toxicity to individuals allows effective prediction of population fate in contaminated environments.

What is needed is more effort to clearly articulate a new population-based paradigm. Also, nontraditional methods must be explored carefully in order to generate a belt of auxiliary hypotheses around this new population-based paradigm. Since the early 1980s (e.g. Moriarty 1983), the argument for population-based methods taking precedence over individual-based metrics of effect has been voiced with increasing frequency in scientific publications, regulatory documents, and federal legislation. Recently, Forbes and Calow (1999) reiterated this theme and provided more evidence to support it by comparing individual- and population-based metrics for ecological impact assessment. Also, individual-based models for populations (e.g. DeAngelis and Gross 1992) have emerged to bridge the gap between individual- and population-based metrics for judging ecological risk.

4.1.2 EVIDENCE SUPPORTING THE NEED FOR THE POPULATION-BASED PARADIGM FOR RISK

The quotes below are chosen to reflect the transition taking place in our thinking about ecotoxicological risk assessment. Notice that early quotes point to the underutilization of population-based metrics of toxicant effect. The need for more population-based predictions is then expressed in a series of regulation-oriented publications. Finally, statements made during the last few years show that methods are now available and are being applied with increasing frequency to address population-level questions.

Ecologists have used the life table since its introduction by Birch (1948) to assess survival, fecundity, and growth rate of populations under various environmental conditions. While it has proved a useful tool in analyzing the dynamics of natural populations, the life table approach has not, with few exceptions..., been used as a toxicity bioassay. (Daniels and Allan 1981)

There is an enormous disparity between the types of data available for assessment and the types of responses of ultimate interest. The toxicological data usually have been obtained from short-term toxicity tests performed using standard protocols and test species. In contrast, the effects of concern to ecologists performing assessments are those of long-term exposures on the persistence, abundance, and/or production of populations. (Barnthouse et al. 1987)

Environmental policy decision makers have shifted emphasis from physiological, individual-level to population-level impacts of human activities. This shift has, in turn, spawned the need for models of population-level responses to such insults as contamination by xenobiotic chemicals. (Emlen 1989)

Protecting populations is an explicitly stated goal of several Congressional and Agency mandates and regulations. Thus it is important that ecological risk assessment guidelines focus upon protection and management at the population, community, and ecosystem levels... (EPA 1991)

The Office of Water is required by the Clean Water Act to restore and maintain the biological integrity of the nation's waters and, specifically, to ensure the protection and propagation of a balanced population of fish, shellfish, and wildlife. (Norton et al. 1992)

The translation from a pollutant's effects on individuals to its effects on the population can be accomplished using life-history analysis to calculate the effect on the population's growth rate. (Sibly 1996)

In this chapter, I am concerned with the translation from individuals to populations using demographic models as a link. Individual organisms are born, grow, reproduce and die, and exposure to toxicants alters the risks of these occurrences. The dynamics of populations are determined by the rates of birth, growth, fertility, and mortality that are produced by these individual events....By incorporating individual rates into population models, the population effects of toxicant-induced changes in those rates can be calculated. (Caswell 1996)

Fortunately, traditional population and demographic analyses can be used to predict the possible outcomes of exposure and their probabilities of occurring. Although most toxicity testing methods do not produce information directly amenable to demographic analysis, some ecotoxicologists have begun to design tests and interpret results in this context. (Newman 1998)

Our conclusion is that r [the population growth rate] *is a better measure of responses to toxicants than are individual-level effects, because it integrates potentially complex interactions among life-history traits and provides a more relevant measure of ecological impact.* (Forbes and Calow 1999)

What is needed is a greater understanding of these approaches and their merits, and the resolve to move to this new context. As suggested in the above quote by Caswell (1996), individual-based information can be used to assess population-level effects if individual-based metrics are produced with translation to the population level in mind. Valuable time and effort are wasted if we are not mindful of the need for hierarchical consilience. Sufficient understanding will foster the generation of more population-based data and its eventual application in routine ecological risk assessments. It will also foster the infusion of methods from disciplines such as conservation biology, fisheries and wildlife management, and agriculture that have similar goals and relevant technologies. Toward these ends, this and the next chapter will build a fundamental understanding of population processes. Some supporting detail including methods for fitting data to these models can be found in Newman (1995).

4.2 FUNDAMENTALS OF POPULATION DYNAMICS

4.2.1 GENERAL

Initially, we assume that a population is composed of similar individuals occupying a spatially uniform habitat. Because the qualities of individuals are lost in models with such assumptions, they are often called phenomenological models — models focused on describing a phenomenon but not linked intimately to causal mechanics, i.e. not mechanistic models. Events occurring to individuals such as birth, growth, reproduction, and death are aggregated into summary statistics such as population rate of increase. Exploration of these models fosters an understanding of population behaviors possible under different conditions. However, without details for individuals and inclusion of interactions with other species populations, insights derived from these models should not be confused with certain knowledge. The problem of ecological inference may appear if results are used to imply behavior of individuals. Alternatively, if results were applied to predicting population fate *in a contaminated ecosystem*, problems may arise because an important emergent property might have been overlooked (e.g. see Box 6.1).

Modeled populations can display continuous or discrete growth dynamics depending on the species and habitat characteristics in question. Continuous growth dynamics are anticipated for a species with overlapping generations and discrete growth dynamics are anticipated for species with nonoverlapping generations. Nonoverlapping generations are common for many annual plant or insect populations. Continuous and discrete growth dynamics are described below with differential and difference equations, respectively. Some of the differential models will also be integrated to allow prediction of population size through time.

4.2.2 PROJECTION BASED ON PHENOMENOLOGICAL MODELS: CONTINUOUS GROWTH

The change in size (N) of a population experiencing unrestrained, continuous growth is described by the differential equation

$$\frac{dN}{dt} = bN - dN = (b - d)N = rN \tag{4.1}$$

where r = the intrinsic rate of increase or per capita growth rate. The r parameter is the difference between the overall birth (b) and death (d) rates (Birch 1948). Obviously, population numbers decline if $b < d$ (i.e. $r < 0$) or increase if $b > d$ (i.e. $r > 0$). Integration of equation (4.1) yields equation (4.2) and allows estimation of population size at any time based on r and the initial population size, N_0:

$$N_t = N_0 e^{rt} \tag{4.2}$$

The amount of time required for the population to double (population doubling time, t_d) is $(\ln 2)/r$.

This model may be applicable for some situations such as the early growth dynamics of a population introduced into a new habitat or a *Daphnia magna* population maintained in a laboratory culture with frequent media replacement. However, most habitats have a finite capacity to sustain the population. This finite capacity slowly comes to have an increasingly important role in the growth dynamics as the population size increases. The change in number of individuals through time slows as the population size approaches the maximum size sustainable by the habitat (the carrying capacity or K). This occurs because b-d is not constant through time. Birth and death rates change as population size increases. More than 150 years ago, Verhulst (1838) accommodated this density-dependence with the term $1 - (N/K)$, producing the logistic model for population density-dependent growth:

$$\frac{dN}{dt} = rN \left(1 - \frac{N}{K} \right) \tag{4.3}$$

The per capita growth rate ($r_{dd} = r(1 - (N/K))$) is now dependent on the population density. As population size increases, birth rates decrease and death rates increase. These rates are $b = b_0 - k_b N$ and $d = d_0 + k_d N$ where b_0 and d_0 are the nearly density-independent birth and deaths rates experienced at very low population densities. The terms, k_b and k_d are slopes for the change in birth and death rates with change in population density. The logistic model can be expressed in these terms (Wilson and Bossert 1971):

$$\frac{dN}{dt} = [(b_0 - k_b N) - (d_0 + k_d N)]N \tag{4.4}$$

The carrying capacity (K) can also be expressed by

$$K = \frac{b_0 - d_0}{k_b + k_d}$$

(Wilson and Bossert 1971).

The model described by equation (4.3) assumes that there is no delay in population response, i.e. there is an instantaneous change in r_{dd} due to any change in density. A delay (T) can be added to equation (4.3) if this is an unreasonable assumption:

$$\frac{dN}{dt} = rN\left(1 - \frac{N_{t-T}}{K}\right) \tag{4.5}$$

A time lag (g) before the population responds favorably to a decrease in density can also be included. Such a lag might be applied for species populations in which individuals must reach a certain age before they are sexually mature:

$$\frac{dN}{dt} = rN_{t-g}\left(1 - \frac{N_{t-T}}{K}\right) \tag{4.6}$$

Gilpin and Ayala (1973) found that the shape of the logistic model was not always the same for different populations and added a term (θ) to equation (4.3) to make the logistic model more flexible. This flexible model (equation (4.7)) is called the θ-logistic model (Figure 4.1):

$$\frac{dN}{dt} = rN\left[1 - \left(\frac{N}{K}\right)^{\theta}\right] \tag{4.7}$$

Obviously, delays could be placed into equation (4.7) if necessary to produce a model of density-dependent growth for a population with time lags in responding to density changes, continuous growth, and a growth symmetry defined by θ.

A density-independent effect (I) on population growth such as that of a toxicant can be added to equation (4.3):

$$\frac{dN}{dt} = rN\left(1 - \frac{N}{K}\right) - I \tag{4.8}$$

The I can also be expressed as some toxicant-related 'loss', 'take', or 'yield' from the population at any moment $(E_{toxicant}N)$ where $E_{toxicant}$ is the proportion

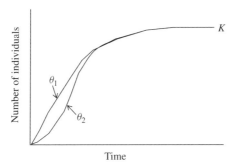

Fig. 4.1. Logistic increase with population growth symmetry being influenced by the θ parameter in the θ-Ricker model (equation (4.7))

of the existing number of individuals (N) taken due to toxicant exposure:

$$\frac{dN}{dt} = rN\left(1 - \frac{N}{K}\right) - E_{\text{Toxicant}}N \tag{4.9}$$

In words, this model predicts the change in number of individuals per unit of time as a function of the intrinsic rate of increase, density-dependent growth dynamics, and a density-independent decrease in numbers of individuals as a result of toxicant exposure. In this form, it is identical to a rudimentary harvesting model for natural populations (e.g. commercial fish harvesting) and is amenable to analysis of population sustainability and recovery (see Everhart, Eipper and Youngs 1953; Gulland 1977; Murray 1993). The difference is that harvesting involves toxicant action instead of fishing. We will discuss this point later but it is important now to realize that toxicant-induced changes in K, r, T, g, and θ are possible and none of these parameters should be ignored in the analysis of population fate with toxicant exposure. If necessary to produce a realistic model, time delays and θ values can be added to equation (4.8). The underlying processes resulting in these delays could be influenced by toxicant exposure. For example, a toxicant may influence the time required for an individual to reach sexual maturity (Chapter 6).

Prediction of population size through time for density-dependent growth of a population with continuous growth dynamics and no time delays is usually done using equations (4.10) or (4.11). These equations are different forms of the sigmoidal growth model. May and Oster (1976) provide other useful forms.

$$N_t = \frac{N_0 K e^{rt}}{K + N_0(e^{rt} - 1)} \tag{4.10}$$

$$N_t = \frac{K}{1 + \left[\dfrac{K - N_0}{N_0}\right] e^{-rt}} \tag{4.11}$$

Newman (1995) describes methods for fitting data to these differential and integrated equations, and relates them to ecotoxicology.

4.2.3 PROJECTION BASED ON PHENOMENOLOGICAL MODELS: DISCRETE GROWTH

Unrestrained growth of populations displaying discrete growth (nonoverlapping generations) is described with the difference equation,

$$N_{t+1} = \lambda N_t \qquad (4.12)$$

where N_t and N_{t+1} are the population sizes at times t and $t + 1$ respectively, and λ is the finite rate of increase which can be related to r (intrinsic or infinitesimal rate of increase) with equation (4.13). It is the number of times that the population multiplies in a time unit or step (Birch 1948). The time step may be arbitrary (e.g. time between census episodes) or associated with some aspect of reproduction (e.g. time between annual calvings):

$$\lambda = \frac{N_{t+1}}{N_t} = e^r \qquad (4.13)$$

The characteristic return time (T_r) can be estimated from r or λ. It is the estimated time required for a population changing in size through time to return toward its carrying capacity or, more generally, toward its steady-state number of individuals (May *et al.* 1974). It is the inverse of the instantaneous growth rate, r, i.e. $T_r = 1/r$. The T_r gets shorter as the growth rate, r, increases: faster growth results in a faster approach toward steady state. In Section 4.4., the influence of T_r on population stability will be described.

This difference equation (equation (4.12)) can be expanded to include density-dependence using several models (see Newman 1995). Equations (4.14) and (4.15) are the classic Ricker and a modification of it that includes Gilpin's θ parameter (the θ-Ricker model), respectively:

$$N_{t+1} = N_t e^{r[1-N_t/K]} \qquad (4.14)$$

$$N_{t+1} = N_t e^{r[1-(N_t/K)^\theta]} \qquad (4.15)$$

As done with the differential models, we have accommodated differences in growth curve symmetry by including a θ term in equation (4.15). But what about adding lag terms? Because the form of the difference equations implies an inherent lag from t to $t + 1$, these models may not need additional terms to accommodate lags. If a lag time different from the time step (t to $t + 1$) is required, it can be added by using N_{t-1}, N_{t-2}, or some other past population size instead of N_t where appropriate in these models. We can add an effect of a density-independent factor such as toxicant exposure to the logistic model. The difference models above are modified by inserting an I term as done in equations (4.8) and (4.9).

The modification made by Newman and Jagoe (1998) to the simplest difference model (equation (4.16)) is provided below (equations (4.17) and (4.18)).

$$N_{t+1} = N_t \left[1 + r \left(1 - \frac{N_t}{K} \right) \right] \tag{4.16}$$

$$N_{t+1} = N_t \left[1 + r \left(1 - \frac{N_t}{K} \right) \right] - I \tag{4.17}$$

$$N_{t+1} = N_t \left[1 + r \left(1 - \frac{N_t}{K} \right) \right] - E_{\text{Toxicant}} N_t \tag{4.18}$$

where I is the number of individuals 'taken' from the parental population by the toxicant at each time step. Again, these models of toxicant effect are comparable to those used to manage harvested, renewable resources such as a fishery. Alternately, Gard (1992) expresses the influence of a toxicant directly in terms of the instantaneous growth rate (r) at time, t:

$$r_t = r_0 - r_1 C_{T(t)} \tag{4.19}$$

where r_0 is the intrinsic rate of increase in the absence of toxicant, $C_{T(t)}$ is a time-dependent effect of the toxicant on the population, and r_1 is a units conversion parameter. Gard's model is composed of three differential equations that link temporal changes in environmental concentrations of a toxicant, concentrations in the organism, and population growth (Gard 1990). At this point, it is only necessary to note that Gard's equations reduce r directly as a consequence of toxicant exposure. Any change in r can influence population stability as we will see in Section 4.3.

4.2.4 SUSTAINABLE HARVEST AND TIME TO RECOVERY

The expressions of toxicant-impacted population growth described to this point are equivalent to those general models explored by Murray (1993) for population harvesting. Therefore, his expansion of associated mathematics and explanations are translated directly in this section into terms of toxicant effects on populations. Let's assume that natality is not affected but the loss of individuals from the population is affected by toxicant exposure. For the differential model (equations (4.8) and (4.9)), Murray defines a harvest or yield that is analogous to I in equation (4.8) and a corresponding new steady-state population size of N_h. This harvest is equivalent to $E \cdot N$ where E is a measure of the harvesting intensity and N is the size of the population being harvested. The E is identical by intent to E_{Toxicant} in equation (4.9). With 'harvesting' or loss upon toxicant exposure, the population will not have a steady-state size of K. Instead, it will have the following steady-state size if r is larger than E_{Toxicant}:

$$N_L = K \left[1 - \frac{E_{\text{Toxicant}}}{r} \right] \tag{4.20}$$

where N_L is equivalent to Murray's N_h except that loss is now due to toxicant exposure. From equation (4.20) it is clear that the population at steady state will drop to 0 if the intensity of the toxicant effect ($E_{Toxicant}$) is equal to or greater than r.

Let's extend Murray's expression of yield from a harvested population in order to gain further insight into the loss that a population can sustain from toxicant exposure without being irreparably damaged. The yield in Murray's equation (1.43) is modified to equation (4.21) in order to define the loss of individuals (L) expected at a certain intensity of effect ($E_{Toxicant}$):

$$L_{E_{Toxicant}} = E_{Toxicant}K\left[1 - \frac{E_{Toxicant}}{r}\right] \tag{4.21}$$

In words, the population loss or 'yield' due to toxicant exposure ($L_{E_{Toxicant}}$) is the new carrying capacity (N_L) multiplied by the $E_{Toxicant}$: the yield is the number of individuals available to be taken times the toxicant-induced fraction 'taken'. Applying equation (4.21), $rK/4$ is the maximum sustainable loss to toxicant exposure (analogous to the maximum sustainable yield where $E_{Toxicant} = r/2$). The new steady-state population size (N_L, equivalent to N_h) will be $K/2$ at this point of maximum sustainable loss or 'yield'. The population is growing maximally under these conditions. Population growth becomes suboptimal if $E_{Toxicant}$ increases further and may even become negative if $E_{Toxicant}$ exceeds r. Figure 4.2 illustrates this general estimation of toxic take or loss for a hypothetical population that is growing according to the logistic model.

Moriarty (1983) makes several important points regarding this approach to analyzing toxicant effects on populations. First, growth measured as a change in number between times t and $t + 1$ will not necessarily decrease with increasing loss from the population due to toxicant exposure. It might increase. Surplus young produced in populations allows a certain level of mortality without an adverse affect on population viability. Different populations have characteristic ranges of loss that can be accommodated. Low losses potentially increase the rate at which new individuals appear in a population and high losses push the population toward local extinction. Second, the carrying capacity of the population will decrease as losses due to toxicant exposure increase. Third, there can be two population sizes that produce a particular yield on either side of the N_t for maximum yield (Figure 4.2). Increases or decreases in toxicant exposure can produce the same results in the context of population change. Failure to recognize this possibility could lead to muddled interpretation of results from monitoring of populations in contaminated habitats. An important advantage of the sustainable yield context just developed is a more complete understanding of population consequences at various intensities of loss due to toxicant exposure.

There is another advantage to ecotoxicologists taking an approach used by renewable resource managers. Often, ecological risk assessments focus on recreational or commercial species, e.g. consequences of toxicant exposure to a salmon

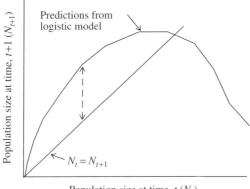

Fig. 4.2. The maximum sustainable yield can be visualized by comparing the curve for the population size at time steps N_t and N_{t+1} to the line for $N_t = N_{t+1}$. The population is not changing from one time to another along the line for $N_t = N_{t+1}$, i.e. the population is at steady state. The vertical distance between the curve of population size at time steps N_t and N_{t+1} and the line for $N_t = N_{t+1}$ defines the sustainable yield resulting from surplus production in the population each time step. The vertical dashed line shows the yield that is maximal for this population. The reader is encouraged to review Waller *et al.* (1971) as an example of using this type of curve with zinc-exposed fathead minnow (*Pimephales promelas*) populations. (Modified from Figure 2.11 of Moriarty 1983 and Figure 2.2a of Murray 1993)

or blue crab fishery. Expressing toxicant effects to populations with the same equations used by fishery or wildlife managers attempting to regulate annual harvest allows simultaneous consideration of losses from human and pollutant 'taking'.

Another characteristic of harvested populations that is useful to the ecotoxicologist is the time to recovery. The time to recover (return to an original population size) after harvest can be estimated in terms of loss due to toxicant exposure. The time to recover (T_R) will increase as E_{Toxicant} increases. This follows from our discussion that characteristic return time decreases as r increases and that E_{Toxicant} has the opposite effect on population growth rate as r. Figure 4.3 shows the general shape of this relationship for a logistic growth model.

The phenomenological models described to this point might have to be modified if interest shifts to smaller and smaller population sizes. Just as a population has a maximum population size (e.g. K), it can also have a minimum population size. The population fails below this minimum number, e.g. the smallest number of individuals in a dispersed population needed to have a chance of sufficient mating and reproductive success, or the minimum number of a social species needed to maintain a viable group. This minimum population size (M) can be

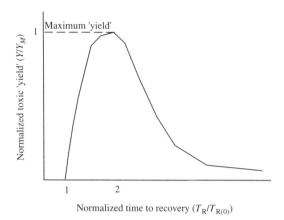

Normalized time to recovery $(T_R/T_{R(0)})$

Fig. 4.3. The time to recover (T_R) will increase as the 'yield' or 'take' due to toxicant exposure $(E_{Toxicant})$ increases. This modification of Figure 1.16a in Murray (1993) shows the general shape of this relationship for a logistic growth model. The $T_{R(0)}$ is the theoretical recovery time in the absence of toxicant exposure $(T_{R(0)} = 1/r)$ and T_R is the recovery time at a particular yield, Y, for the steady-state population. Yield is normalized in this figure by dividing it by the maximum possible yield (Y_M)

placed into the logistic model (equation (4.3)) (Wilson and Bossert 1971):

$$\frac{dN}{dt} = rN \left(1 - \frac{N}{K}\right)\left(1 - \frac{M}{N}\right) \tag{4.22}$$

The population will go locally extinct if N falls below M.

More discussion of population loss, recovery time, and minimum population size in the context of fishery management can be found in books by Gulland (1977) and Everhart, Eipper and Youngs (1953), and formulations relative to discrete growth models are provided in Murray (1993). Because some fisheries models based on commercial yield consider monetary costs, the application of a common model also provides an opportunity in risk management decisions to integrate monetary gain from fishing with monetary loss due to toxicant exposure. A management failure of a fishery would certainly occur if, by ignoring toxicant effects, one optimized based solely on commercial fishery harvest. Perhaps the additional loss due to toxicant exposure would put the combined consequences to the population beyond the optimal yield and the fishery would slowly begin an inexplicable decline.

4.3 POPULATION STABILITY

Until approximately 25 years ago, the dynamics in population size described by models such as equations (4.3), (4.14), and (4.16) were thought to consist of an

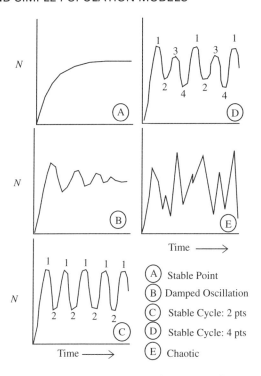

Fig. 4.4. Temporal dynamics that might arise from the differential and difference models of population growth

increase to some steady-state size (e.g. K) as depicted in Figure 4.1. Deviations from this monotonic increase toward K were attributed to random processes. In 1974, Robert May published a remarkably straightforward paper in *Science* demonstrating that this was not the complete story. Even the simple models described in this chapter can display complex oscillations in population size and, at an extreme, chaotic dynamics. Some populations do monotonically increase to a steady-state size (i.e. Stable Point in Figure 4.4). Others tend to overshoot the carrying capacity, turn to oscillate back and forth around the carrying capacity, and eventually settle down to the carrying capacity (i.e. Damped Oscillation in Figure 4.4). Sizes of other populations oscillate indefinitely around the carrying capacity (i.e. Stable Cycles in Figure 4.4). These oscillations may be between 2, 4, 8, 16 or more points. Beyond population conditions resulting in stable oscillations, the number of individuals in a population at any time may be best defined as chaotic (Chaotic in Figure 4.4). Population size changes in an unpredictable fashion through time. The exact size at any time is very dependent on the initial conditions: on average, trajectories for populations with slightly differing initial sizes separate exponentially through time (Schaffer and Kot 1986). Although chaotic dynamics have been noted for only a few species populations (e.g. flour beetles, *Tribolium castaneum* (Costantino *et al*. 1997)), these complex population dynamics are fostered by high r, long time lags, and periodic forcing functions like those used to model impacts of weather extremes or insecticide spraying of target populations. There is no reason to reject the notion that nontarget species with high rates of increase and/or significant time lags that live near agricultural fields might exhibit chaotic dynamics.

What specific qualities determine a population's growth dynamics? The dynamics tend to move from stable point to damped oscillations to stable cycles to chaotic dynamics as the intrinsic rate of increase (r), time lag (T), and/or θ increase. The rate at which population size approaches K increases as the r increases: at a certain r, the population tends to overshoot K and move the temporal dynamics into more complicated oscillations. Similarly, if the time lag (T) increases, the populations size begins to oscillate more and more as the population tends to over- and then undershoot the carrying capacity. The exact conditions producing these different dynamics (i.e. the stability regions) have been determined for several of the simple models described in this chapter. Table 4.1 provides those for equations (4.5) and (4.14)–(4.16). The derivation of these stability criteria is detailed in May *et al*. (1974). May (1976a,b) extends the graphical approach used in Figure 4.2 to show the conditions leading to different population dynamics.

Several points relevant to population ecotoxicology emerge from these considerations of population dynamics. During an ecological risk assessment, the population size at a contaminated site might be compared to that of a reference site. The observation of a smaller population at the contaminated site relative to the uncontaminated site often leads to the conclusion of an adverse effect on the population. As demonstrated by the models above, some populations will characteristically have wide variations in size through time. Others will be more stable. To compare sizes of populations from reference and contaminated sites using data from one or a few field samplings can lead to invalid conclusions if populations at both sites normally display wide oscillations. Additionally, because toxicants can affect r, T and θ in these simple models, there is no reason to believe that toxicants will not impact population dynamics. Therefore, it may be important to consider pollutant effects on population dynamics in addition to population size. The likelihood of a local population extinction is greatly increased by a toxicant exposure that produces wide oscillations in addition to lowering the population-carrying capacity. The lowering of the carrying capacity brings the population numbers closer to the minimal population number (M) and the oscillation troughs periodically bring the population numbers even closer to M.

Higher-order interactions are also possible on population dynamics. Simkiss, Daniels and Smith (1993) examined the growth of blowfly (*Lucilia sericata*) under different combinations of food and cadmium. Food deprivation and cadmium concentration were additive in their effects on key growth components

Table 4.1. Stability regions for differential (equation (4.5)) and difference (equations (4.15), (4.14) and (4.16)) models of population growth

Stability region	Differential	Difference equations		
	Equation (4.5)	Equation (4.15)	Equation (4.14)	Equation (4.16)
Stable Point	$0 < rT < e^{-1}$	$0 < r\theta < 1$	$2 > r > 0$	$2 > r > 0$
Damped Oscillation	$e^{-1} < rT < 0.5\pi$	$1 < r\theta < 2$		
Stable Cycles	$0.5_{\pi < rT}$	$2 < r\theta < 2.69$		
Between 2 points			$2.526 > r > 2.000$	$2.449 > r > 2.000$
Between 4 points			$2.656 > r > 2.526$	$2.544 > r > 2.449$
Between 8 points			$2.685 > r > 2.656$	$2.564 > r > 2.544$
Between 16 or more points			$2.692 > r > 2.685$	$2.570 > r > 2.564$
Chaotic dynamics		$2.69 < r\theta$	$r > 2.692$	$r > 2.570$

Stability region information for equations (4.5), (4.15), (4.14), (4.16) was obtained from May (1976a,b), Thomas, Pomerantz and Gilpin (1980), May (1974) and May (1974), respectively.

(maximum larval size, development period, pupal weight, adult weight at emergence, and fecundity). Many of these effects change r and time lags. Therefore, the combination of cadmium exposure and limited food availability can influence population dynamics. Nicholson (1954) had previously shown that limited food alone produced population oscillations with *Lucilia cuprina*. Simkiss, Daniels and Smith (1993) predicted from their studies of food and cadmium effects on blowfly populations that 'sublethal levels of cadmium might therefore lead to smaller-amplitude fluctuations without affecting the mean population level'.

Box 4.1 Extinction probabilities for fruit fly populations under nutritional stress

The influence of environmental carrying capacity on the likelihood of *Drosophila* sp. population extinction was quantified by Philippi *et al.* (1987) by manipulating the amount of food available to cultures of different fruit fly species. In one set of experiments, food was varied from a very restrictive 3 ml per 120 ml bottle to an excessive amount of 40 ml per 120 ml bottle. Flies were periodically transferred to new bottles of media and the results were fit to a difference logistic model that included Gilpin's θ parameter:

$$\Delta N = N_{t+1} - N_t = rN_t - \frac{r}{K^\theta}N_t^{(\theta+1)} \tag{4.23}$$

The premise was that, as they had seen with species populations competing with one another for limited resources, isolated fly populations provided with limited resources would exhibit very wide fluctuations in size. These fluctuations would increase the chance of population extinction. In a second set of experiments, they varied the density of flies, and measured survival and reproduction of individuals at these different densities. The resulting data were used to assess the relative contributions of chaotic dynamics, carrying capacity reduction, and environmental stochasticity to population persistence.

Let's assume in interpreting their results for nutritional stress that, according to equations (4.9), (4.18) and (4.20) and the work of Simkiss *et al.* (1993), toxicant exposure will similarly impact fruit fly populations by decreasing carrying capacity. Under this assumption, this study of food limitation has direct relevance to populations exposed to toxicants.

Much to their surprise, the food-deprived populations showed lower variability than those with unlimited food: the stressed populations had reduced variability in their numbers. Higher observed rates of extinction in food-deprived populations were a result of a reduced carrying capacity and variance in growth dynamics due to environmental variability, not a shift toward more complicated dynamics. (The stability regions for this θ-logistic model are those given for equation (4.15) in Table 4.1.) The environmental variability involved differences in the amount of food placed into each bottle, the humidity, and level of bacterial contamination introduced into cultures during handling. They conclude that the minimum viable population size (M) is determined by deterministic and stochastic population processes but, in this case, a deterministic shift in population dynamics toward wider fluctuations under stressful conditions was not responsible for the observed accelerated rates of extinction.

Sensitivity analysis for the model provided further insight into the relative importance of changes in r and θ on the probability of population extinction. Simulations demonstrated that extinction probabilities over a wide range of r and θ values were determined by chaotic dynamics regardless of the level of environmental noise only if $r \cdot \theta$ was greater than 3. At the other extreme, systems with low r and θ values (i.e. those that we are assuming would be characteristic of pollutant-stressed populations), recover very slowly from minor perturbations. In this situation, extinction probability increases with environmental variability. The lowest probabilities of extinction were in regions with $0.5 < r \cdot \theta < 2$.

4.4 SPATIAL DISTRIBUTIONS OF INDIVIDUALS IN POPULATIONS

In Section 4.2, the convenient assumption was made that a population is composed of similar individuals occupying a spatially uniform habitat. However, individuals are often distributed heterogeneously within a habitat that may not be homogeneous itself. Some consequences of this heterogeneity will be outlined in this section.

4.4.1 DESCRIBING DISTRIBUTIONS: CLUMPED, RANDOM AND UNIFORM

Individuals may be distributed uniformly, randomly, or in clusters within a habitat (Figure 4.5). Uniform distributions are rare. The most obvious, and especially trivial, example of a population with a uniform distribution of individuals is a silvacultural plantation. Random distributions are much more common. Clumped or aggregated populations are also common. The driving force for the clumping may be innate to the species (e.g. the social gathering of individuals to enhance foraging or reproductive success), result from extrinsic factors (e.g. a landscape that is a mosaic of widely differing areas of habitat quality), or emerge from an interaction of intrinsic and extrinsic factors.

The conformity of individuals within a population to these patterns can be formally tested by methods described in various sources (i.e, Krebs 1989; Ludwig and Reynolds 1988; Newman 1995) by assuming that positive binomial, Poisson, and negative binomial models describe uniform, random, and clumped patterns,

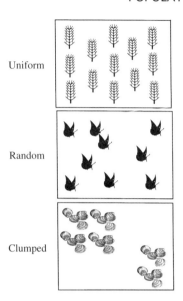

Fig. 4.5. General distributional patterns of individuals within populations including uniform (top panel), random (middle panel), and clumped (bottom panel) distributions

respectively. These models can also be fit to distributional data for individuals using methods described in the cited sources.

4.4.2 METAPOPULATIONS

What are the consequences of an uneven distribution of individuals within a habitat? Do things simply average out over the entire habitat and, as a consequence, generally conform to the simple population dynamics described so far? The simple answer is no. Unique and important qualities emerge in the dynamics and persistence of a metapopulation. Hanski (1996) described a metapopulation as 'a set of local populations which interact via dispersing individuals among local populations; though not all local populations in a metapopulation interact, directly with every other local population'. Unique qualities of metapopulations must be understood in order to appreciate the influence of toxicant exposure on populations.

4.4.2.1 Metapopulation Dynamics

Subpopulations or local populations can occupy patches of the available habitat that differ slightly or greatly relative to the ability to foster individual survival, growth, and reproduction. Consequently, individual fitnesses differ among landscape patches. High-quality patches may produce so many individuals that they act as sources to other patches. Low-quality patches may be so inferior that they do not produce surplus individuals. To remain occupied, inferior sink subpopulations rely on an influx of individuals from source patches. Some patches may be so superior relative to other marginal patches that they are keystone habitats (O'Connor 1996) without which the metapopulation might disappear. Which patches are sources and which are sinks may change through time depending on factors like weather, disease, competition, or predation pressures In other situations, patches are physical islands and the source–sink structure will remain stable through time. A source–sink dynamic emerges as essential in understanding metapopulation size and persistence on the landscape scale (Figure 4.6).

Levins (1969, 1970; cited in Hanski 1996) explored metapopulation dynamics with a simple model:

$$\frac{dp}{dt} = mp(1 - p) - ep \qquad (4.24)$$

where p is the size of the metapopulation expressed as the proportion of available patches that are occupied, e is the rate or probability of extinction in patches and m is the rate or probability of population reappearance in (or immigration

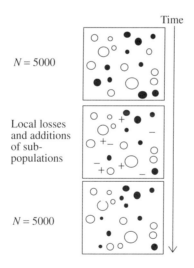

Fig. 4.6. Stable metapopulation dynamics within a habitat mosaic despite periodic local extinctions. Subpopulations vary in their ability to act as sources (size of open circles) and sinks (size of filled circle), resulting in different probabilities of local extinction through time (top panel). Because of the exchange among patches, the metapopulation persists through a dynamic steady state of extinctions (− in middle panel) and reestablishments via influx from nearby sources. New populations are also established through time via influx from sources (+ in middle panel). The net result is metapopulation persistence through time (bottom panel)

into) vacant patches of the landscape mosaic. In more general terms, this model says that the $\mathrm{d}p/\mathrm{d}t$ is the difference between the immigration rate and the extinction rate for patches in a habitat mosaic (Gotelli 1991). The probability of patch extinction is independent of the regional occurrence of subpopulations (p): the likelihood of a patch being vacated is not influenced by the proportion of nearby patches that are occupied. As we will see in a moment, this may or may not be a good assumption. This model can be modified into a form analogous to the logistic model for population size 'with m-e being the intrinsic rate of metapopulation increase for a small metapopulation (when p is small), while $1 - e/m$ is the equivalent of the local 'carrying capacity', the stable equilibrium point toward which p moves in time' (Hanski 1996):

$$
\frac{\mathrm{d}p}{\mathrm{d}t} = (m - e)p \left(1 - \frac{p}{1 - \frac{e}{m}} \right)
\tag{4.25}
$$

(*Note*: This model has conceptual similarities to the MacArthur–Wilson model for island colonization of species.)

Gotelli (1991) provides more detail for this and related metapopulation models. He also highlights several themes in metapopulation dynamics. First, he describes the rescue effect as the lowering of the probability of patch extinction because of the influx of individuals from nearby subpopulations, i.e. the assumption in equation (4.25) is avoided that the probability of patch extinction is independent of the regional occurrence of populations (p). The model of Hanski (described in Gotelli 1991) includes the rescue effect by slight modification of equation (4.24) to equation (4.26). In this model, the probability of local extinction decreases as p (proportion of patches occupied) increases: emigration from neighboring subpopulations reduces the likelihood of local extinction:

$$
\frac{\mathrm{d}p}{\mathrm{d}t} = mp(1 - p) - ep(1 - p)
\tag{4.26}
$$

In equation (4.24), the extinction rate increases as p increases. In equation (4.26), this is true up to a certain p. The extinction rate then begins to decline as p continues to increase.

A source of propagules such as a seed bank or dormant stage can produce a 'propagule rain' that bolsters a waning subpopulation and can influence metapopulation dynamics. In this case, the regional occurrence of subpopulations (p) does not impact the rate of reappearance of individuals (m) and the rain of propagules increases the m by $m(1 - p)^2$ (Gotelli 1991). Under this condition and an e that is independent of regional occurrence, a better description of metapopulation dynamics is as follows (Gotelli 1991):

$$\frac{dp}{dt} = m(1 - p) - ep \qquad (4.27)$$

Equation (4.28) combines the propagule rain and rescue effects:

$$\frac{dp}{dt} = m(1 - p) - ep(1 - p) \qquad (4.28)$$

Additional details and examples can be obtained in Lewin (1989), Gotelli (1991), Gilpin and Hanski (1991), Pulliam and Danielson (1991), Hanski (1996), and Pulliam (1996). O'Connor (1996) reviews metapopulation consequences of toxicant exposure.

4.4.2.2 Consequences to Exposed Populations

The paradigms of landscape ecology and metapopulation dynamics...have introduced new concepts of spatial dynamics whose implications for ecological risk assessment have only just begun to receive attention. (O'Connor 1996)

The metapopulation context is quickly being incorporated into conservation biology efforts but is only slowly being considered in ecotoxicology. Regardless, several consequences become obvious from this brief sketch of metapopulation dynamics. First, a rudimentary assessment of population status in a contaminated area requires consideration of adjacent subpopulations, otherwise observations might be inexplicable. Perhaps toxicity tests suggest that a species should be absent from a contaminated site but the presence of a source population produces an apparently thriving population on the site, i.e. the rescue effect. Second, if the lost habitat was a keystone habitat, the population consequences will be much worse than suggested by any narrow assessment based on the percentage of total habitat lost. Third, the creation of corridors to enhance movement among patches could be more beneficial in some cases than complete removal of contaminated media from a site. Indeed, remediation often causes massive disruption of habitat: a thoughtful balance in removal of polluted media from patches, creation of corridors among patches, and building of barriers around other highly contaminated patches could result in optimal remediation. Fourth, among migrating individuals within the mosaic of habitats, some will have spent time in heavily contaminated patches. The result might be that individuals exposed in one patch will have their population-level consequences manifested in a subpopulation removed from that contaminated site. Spromberg, John and Mandis (1998) call this the effect at a distance hypothesis because the action of a toxicant exposure occurs at a place spatially distant from the contamination. Fifth, a sublethal effect that reduces migration-related behavior could decrease the stability or persistence of a metapopulation by affecting the rate at which vacant habitat is refilled from adjacent areas.

Box 4.2   Computer projections of metapopulation risk in a contaminated habitat

Spromberg, John and Mandis (1998) developed phenomenological models for subpopulations in a habitat with patchy distributions of individuals and toxicants. Their intent was to explore consequences of such a metapopulation configuration and to relate the results to risk-assessment activities and possible remedial actions. They described their conceptual framework with equations (4.24) and (4.26) above, and added the diffusion reaction model of Wu, Vankat and Barlas (1993):

$$\frac{dN_i}{dt} = N_i f(N_i) + \sum_{j=i} [d_{ij}(N_j - N_i)] \tag{4.29}$$

where d_{ij} is the migration rate from patch i to patch j, N_i and N_j are the number of individuals in patches i and j, respectively, and $f()$ is a function of N that defines the population growth rate. Note that, unlike previous models, the numbers of individuals in the patches is being modeled in equation (4.29), not the proportion of all patches that are occupied (p).

Equation (4.29) is used to simulate the dynamics of a metapopulation under different contamination scenarios involving three patches (Figure 4.7). Simulations included a contaminant that quickly disappeared from a patch (e.g. a quickly degraded pesticide) and a persistent contaminant. The model assumed the following: (1) density-dependent growth, (2) density-dependent patch immigration and emigration, and (3) distance-dependent movement of individuals between patches. As an example of distant-dependent movement among patches, the distance between all three patches were similar for the model in the top panel of Figure 4.7, but the distance between the two outer patches in the model at the bottom of this figure was twice as far as the distance from any one of these outer patches to the center patch. For the model in the bottom panel, the distance-dependent movement between an outer patch and the central one was much higher than the movement between the two outside patches. Computation of migration rate from patch i to j was done with the simple equation, $d_{ij} = (N_i H_j)/D_{ij}$, where H_j is the habitat available to be occupied in patch j and D_{ij} is the distance between the two patches.

Other model assumptions included a constant carrying capacity and minimum population size for a patch, no avoidance of contaminated habitat, no compensatory reproduction due to the presence of toxicant, a Poisson distribution to define the probability of an individual being exposed to a toxicant in the contaminated patch, constant bioavailability of toxicant, and the occurrence of no other stochastic disturbances, e.g. no weather-related mortalities.

The results of the simulations are easily summarized. A toxic effect can be seen in subpopulations of nearby, uncontaminated patches due to the movement of individuals into those patches from a contaminated patch. Again, the

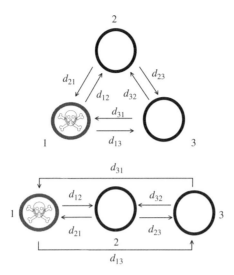

Fig. 4.7. The three patch metapopulations simulated by Spromberg, John and Mandis (1998). Patches with skull and crossbones indicate contaminated patches and the open symbol represents uncontaminated patches. As described in the text, d_{ij} indicates the migration rate from patch i to patch j. Modified from Figure 1 of Spromberg, John and Mandis (1998)

authors refer to this as the hypothesis of effect at distance. Toxicant-induced reduction in subpopulation size in one patch results in a higher rate of movement of individuals into that patch. In the model in the bottom panel of Figure 4.7, even 100% mortality in the contaminated patch does not produce a local extinction. Individuals move into the vacated patch from the other patches. One noteworthy conclusion derived from the simulations was that a reference population picked from near a contaminated site might not produce useful information in an ecological risk assessment. Although not contaminated, the subpopulation occupying that clean patch may still be impacted by the toxicant due to migration of individuals from the contaminated patch. Conversely, remediation of a site can result in improvements in population viability in patches outside that containing the toxicant.

4.5 SUMMARY

Population-based assessment endpoints will eventually come to occupy a more central role in ecological risk assessments. To facilitate this change, relevant concepts and methods must be described so that ecotoxicologists feel comfortable with their application. Population-based metrics of effect will need to accumulate in databases such as the AQUIRE database maintained by the US Environmental Protection Agency. Obviously, consilience among levels is essential as the new, population-centered paradigm emerges. Linkage to individual-based effects can be made with individual-based population models such as some of the demographic analyses described in the next chapter. However, data must be collected so that these links can be made. Presently, they often are not collected in an appropriate manner. Linkage to community-level effects is also possible with the context developed in this chapter. For example, the metapopulation formulations (e.g. equation (4.25)) are closely related to the community succession models (MacArthur-Wilson model) used by Cairns *et al.* (1986) to predict toxicant effects to protozoan community processes.

4.5.1 SUMMARY OF FOUNDATION CONCEPTS AND PARADIGMS

- A population-based paradigm for assessing ecological risk should replace the currently reigning paradigm based on metrics for effect to individuals.

- Phenomenological models of population dynamics provide an understanding of possible behaviors of populations, including those experiencing toxicant exposure. However, they do not provide certain knowledge, i.e. perfect prediction.

- Toxicant exposure can change the population qualities reflected in the model parameters, r, λ, K, T, g, T_R, M, and θ.

- Effects of toxicant exposure can be included in conventional growth models as a density-independent loss from the population.

- Toxicant exposure can result in reduced population size.

- Toxicant exposures can change population dynamics.

- Toxicant exposure can result in an increase in the probability of population extinction.

- Population sustainability and recovery with toxicant exposure can be modeled with modifications to methods used to manage harvested, renewable resources such as a commercial or recreational fishery.

- Increased toxicant exposure may not necessarily result in a decrease in population production rate. Populations can lose a number of their surplus offspring without a significant change in population viability. On either side of the maximum sustainable loss to toxicant exposure ('yield') are equal points of excess production by the population. (See Section 4.2.4.)

- Expression of loss due to toxicant exposure in terms used by managers of renewable resources, e.g. commercial fishery managers, allows the integration of toxicant and fishing/harvesting activities in assessments of resource sustainability.

- Temporal dynamics of populations can take several forms including monotonic increase to carrying capacity, damped oscillations to carrying capacity, stable oscillations about carrying capacity, or chaotic dynamics. These dynamics are determined by combinations of r, T, and θ (see Table 4.1). Because r, T, and θ can be changed by toxicant exposure, population dynamics can be changed by toxicant exposure.

- Individuals can be nonrandomly distributed in available habitat. Distribution of individuals in a population can be influenced by innate qualities of the species and/or qualities of the environment, including the presence of toxicants.

- Metapopulation dynamics influence the probability of population extinction in landscape mosaics contaminated with toxicants.

- Habitats have finite, but fluctuating, capacities to support a species population and toxicants can lower (e.g. reduction of amount of food or suitable habitat) or increase (e.g. remove a competitor or predator) the carrying capacity of a habitat.

- Assessment of toxicant exposure consequences to a metapopulation must consider source-sink dynamics, keystone habitats, and the possibilities of the rescue effect and a significant propagule rain effect.

- Creation of corridors between patches or isolation of the contaminated patch may greatly influence population viability. These actions should be considered in addition to conventional removal of contaminated media in remediation plans.

REFERENCES

Barnthouse LW, Suter II GW, Rosen AE and Beauchamp JJ (1987). Estimating responses of fish populations to toxic contaminants. *Environ Toxicol Chem* **6**: 811–824.

Birch LC (1948). The intrinsic rate of natural increase of an insect population. *J An Ecol* **17**: 15–26.

Braithwaite RB (1983). The structure of a scientific system. In *The Concept of Evidence* ed. by R. Achinstein, pp. 44–62, Oxford University Press, Oxford.

Cairns Jr. J, Pratt JR, Niederlehner BR and McCormick PV (1986). A simple cost-effective multispecies toxicity test using organisms with a cosmopolitan distribution. *Environ Monit Assess* **6**: 207–220.

Caswell H (1996). Demography meets ecotoxicology: untangling the population level effects of toxic substances. In *Ecotoxicology. A Hierarchical Treatment*, ed. by MC Newman and CH Jagoe, pp. 255–292, Lewis/CRC Press, Boca Raton, FL.

Costantino, RF, Desharnais RA, Cushing JM and Dennis B (1997). Chaotic dynamics in an insect population. *Science* **275**: 389–391.

Daniels, RE and Allan JD (1981). Life table evaluation of chronic exposure to a pesticide. *Can. J Fish Aquat Sci* **38**: 485–494.

DeAngelis DL and Gross LJ (eds). (1992). *Individual-based Models and Approaches in Ecology*, Chapman & Hall, New York.

Emlen JM (1989). Terrestrial population models for ecological risk assessment: a state-of-the-art review. *Environ Toxicol Chem* **8**: 831–842.

EPA (1991). *Summary Report on Issues in Ecological Risk Assessment, EPA/625/3–91/018* February. NTIS, Springfield, VA.

Everhart WH, Eipper AW and Youngs WD (1953). *Principles of Fishery Science*. Cornell University Press, Ithaca, NY.

Forbes, VE and Calow P (1999). Is the per capita rate of increase a good measure of population-level effects in ecotoxicology? *Environ Toxicol Chem* **18**: 1544–1556.

Gard TC (1990). A stochastic model for the effects of toxicants on populations. *Ecol. Modeling* **51**: 273–280.

Gard TC (1992). Stochastic models for toxicant-stressed populations. *Bull Math Biol* **54**: 827–837.

Gilpin ME and Ayala FJ (1973). Global models of growth and competition. *Proc Natl Acad Sci USA* **70**: 3590–3593.

Gilpin ME and Hanski I (eds) (1991). *Metapopulation Dynamics: Empirical and Theoretical Investigations*. Harcourt Brace Jovanovich, London.

Gotelli NJ (1991). Metapopulation models: the rescue effect, the propagule rain, and the core-satellite hypothesis. *Am Nat* **138**: 768–776.

Gulland JA (1977). *Fish Population Dynamics*. John Wiley, London.

Hanski I (1996). Metapopulation ecology. In *Population Dynamics in Ecological Space and Time*. ed. by OE Rhodes Jr, RK Chesser and MH Smith, The University of Chicago Press, Chicago, IL.

Howson C and Urbach P (1989). *Scientific Reasoning. The Bayesian Approach*, Open Court Publishing Company, La Salle, IL.

Krebs CJ (1989). *Ecological Methodology*. HarperCollins, New York.

Kuhn TS (1962). *The Structure of Scientific Revolutions*, The University of Chicago Press, Chicago, IL.

Lakatos I (1970). Falsification and the methodology of scientific research programmes. In *Criticism and the Growth of Knowledge*, ed. by I Lakatos and A Musgrave, pp. 91–196, Cambridge University Press, Cambridge.

Levins R (1969). Some demographic and genetic consequences of environmental heterogeneity for biological control. *Bull Entomol Soc Am* **15**: 237–240.

Levins R (1970). Extinction.*Lect Math Life Sci* **2**: 75–107.

Lewin R (1989). Sources and sinks complicate ecology. *Science* **243**: 477–478.

Loehle C (1987). Hypothesis testing in ecology. Psychological aspects and the importance of theory maturation. Quart Rev Biol **62**: 397–409.

Ludwig JA and Reynolds JF (1988). *Statistical Ecology. A Primer on Methods and Computing*. John Wiley, New York.

May RM (1974). Biological populations with nonoverlapping generations: stable points, stable cycles, and chaos. *Science* **186**: 645–647.

May RM (1976a). *Theoretical Ecology. Principles and Applications*. WB Saunders Co., Philadelphia, PA.

May RM (1976b). Simple mathematical models with very complicated dynamics. *Nature* **261**: 459–467.

May RM, Conway GR, Hassell MP and Southwood TRE (1974). Time delays, density-dependence and single-species oscillations. *J Anim Ecol* **43**: 747–770.

May RM and Oster GF (1976). Bifurcation and dynamic complexity in simple ecological models. *Am Nat* **110**: 573–599.

Moriarty F (1983). *Ecotoxicology. The Study of Pollutants in Ecosystems*. Academic Press, London.

Murray JD (1993). *Mathematical Biology*. Springer-Verlag, Berlin.

Newman MC (1995). *Quantitative Methods in Aquatic Ecotoxicology*. Lewis/CRC Press, Boca Raton, FL.

Newman MC (1998). *Fundamentals of Ecotoxicology*. Ann Arbor/Lewis/CRC Press, Boca Raton, FL.

Newman MC and Jagoe RH (1998). Allozymes reflect the population-level effect of mercury: simulations of the mosquitofish (*Gambusia holbrooki* Girard) GPI-2 response. *Ecotoxiology* **7**: 141–150.

Nicholson AJ (1954). An outline of the dynamics of animal populations. *Australian J Zool* **2**: 9–65.

Norton SB, Rodier DJ, Gentile JH, Van der Schalie WH, Wood WP and Slimak MW (1992). A framework for ecological risk assessment at the EPA. *Environ Toxicol Chem* **11**: 1663–1672.

O'Connor RJ (1996). Toward the incorporation of spatiotemporal dynamics into ecotoxicology. In *Population Dynamics in Ecological Space and Time*, ed. by OE Rhodes Jr, RK Chesser and MH Smith. The University of Chicago Press, Chicago, IL.

Philippi TE, Carpenter MP, Case TJ and Gilpin ME (1987). *Drosophila* population dynamics: chaos and extinction. *Ecology* **68**: 154–159.

Piatelli-Palmarini M (1994). *Inevitable Illusions*. John Wiley, New York.

Popper KR (1972). *Objective Knowledge. An Evolutionary Approach*. Clarendon Press, Oxford.

Pulliam HR (1996). Sources and sinks: empirical evidence and population consequences. In *Population Dynamics in Ecological Space and Time*, OE Rhodes Jr, RK Chesser and MH Smith. The University of Chicago Press, Chicago, IL.

Pulliam HR and Danielson BJ (1991). Sources, sinks, and habitat selection: a landscape perspective on population dynamics. *Am Nat* **137**: S50–S66.

Schaffer WM and Kot M (1986). Chaos in ecological systems: the coals that Newcastle forgot. *TREE* **1**: 58–63.

Sibly RM (1996). Effects of pollutants on individual life histories and population growth rates. In *Ecotoxicology. A Hierarchical Treatment*. ed. by MC Newman and CH Jagoe. pp. 197–223, Lewis/CRC Press, Boca Raton, FL.

Simkiss K, Daniels S and Smith RH (1993). Effects of population density and cadmium toxicity on growth and survival of blowflies. *Environ Pollut* **81**: 41–45.

Spromberg JA, John BM and Mandis WG (1998). Metapopulation dynamics: indirect effects and multiple distinct outcomes in ecological risk assessment.*Environ Toxicol Chem* **17**: 1640–1649.

Thomas WR, Pomerantz MJ and Gilpin ME (1980). Chaos, asymmetric growth and group selection for dynamical stability. *Ecology* **6**: 1312–1320.

Verhulst PF (1838). Notice sur la loi que la population suit dans son accroissement. *Corr Math et Phys* **10**: 113–121.

Waller WT, Dahlberg ML, Sparks RE and Cairns Jr J (1971). A computer simulation of the effects of superimposed mortality due to pollutants of fathead minnows (*Pimephales promelas*). *J Fish Res Bd Canada* **28**: 1107–1112.

Wilson EO and Bossert WH (1971). *A Primer of Population Biology*. Sinauer Associates, Inc, Sunderland, MA.

Wu J, Vankat JL and Barlas Y (1993). Effects of patch connectivity and arrangement on animal metapopulation dynamics: a simulation study. *Ecol Model* **65**: 221–254.

5 Toxicants and Population Demographics

...there's a special providence in the fall of a sparrow. If it be now, 'tis not to come; if it be not to come, it will be now; if it be not now, yet it will come: the readiness is all ... (Hamlet Act V, Scene II)

5.1 DEMOGRAPHY – ADDING INDIVIDUAL HETEROGENEITY TO POPULATION MODELS

Discussion so far grew from phenomenological models involving identical and uniformly distributed individuals to metapopulation models incorporating spatial heterogeneity. Now demography, the quantitative study of death, birth, age, migration, and sex in populations, will be applied to include age and sex differences among individuals. These important differences among individuals produce distinct vital rates, i.e. rates of death, birth, and migration. Combined, these vital rates determine a population's overall qualities. In fact, population vital rates were aggregated earlier into summary statistics such as the intrinsic rate of increase, resulting in hidden information and imperfect insights. Finally, metapopulation models including demographic vital rates can be formulated to obtain the fullest description of and most realistic predictions of population consequences of toxicant exposure. Variation in vital rates can be added also to render a stochastic model. Such a model could be applied to estimate the probability of local extinction for a metapopulation based on contaminant-induced changes in vital rates.

Despite current convention in ecological risk assessment, demographic analysis is essential to accurately determine the qualities and fate of exposed populations. Present precepts in ecotoxicology suggest that a species population will remain viable if the most sensitive life stage of the species is 'protected', e.g. toxicant concentrations do not exceed the NOEC or MATC concentration for that life stage. Early life stage testing results are applied under the premise that the *population* will remain viable if the weakest link in an *individual's* chain of life stages is protected. But this is not always true. Newman (1998) refers to this false paradigm as the weakest link incongruity. The most sensitive stage of an individual's life cycle might not be the most crucial relative to population vitality or viability (Petersen and Petersen 1988; Kammenga *et al.* 1996). This will become more obvious as we discuss reproductive value and related topics below. Fortunately, ecotoxicology is rapidly moving toward balanced inclusion of demographic analysis (e.g. Daniels and Alan 1981; Münzinger and Guarducci 1988; Pesch, Munns and Gurjahra-Gobell 1991; Martinez-Jerónimo et al. 1993; Bechmann 1994; Koivisto and Ketola 1995). Required now is a sustained and insightful integration of demography into assessments of ecological risk. The intent of this chapter is to contribute to this integration by describing foundation demographic concepts and methods. Straightforward algebraic (e.g. Marshall 1962) and matrix (e.g. Leslie 1945, 1948; Caswell 1996) formulations will be described because both are applied in population ecotoxicology.

5.1.1 STRUCTURED POPULATIONS

Age-, stage-, and sex-dependent vital rates will be considered in this section. Age data may be applied when available. Alternatively, analyses might focus on vital rates at different life stages such as larval → juvenile → adult stages. For example, the effects of dioxin and polychlorinated biphenyls (PCBs) on *Fundulus heteroclitus* populations were modeled by considering the following life stages: embryos → larvae → 28-day larvae → 1-year old adults → 2-year-old adults → 3-year old-adults (Munns et al. 1997). Sex-dependent vital rates can be important too but our focus here will remain primarily on females of differing ages or stages.

5.1.2 BASIC LIFE TABLES

Life tables or schedules are constructed for: mortality alone, both mortality and birth (natality), or mortality, natality and migration combined. By definition, there is no migration to be considered in a closed population but migration may be important in an open one. Obviously, analysis of a metapopulation would obligate the inclusion of movement among subpopulations. In this chapter, we will show calculations relevant to closed populations only; however, inclusion of these methods in metapopulation models would be possible using concepts described in the previous chapter.

Data for life tables can be gathered in three ways. To produce a cohort life table, a cohort of individuals is followed through time with measurement of mortality alone, or mortality and natality. As an example, a group of 1000 young-of-the-year may be tagged during the calving season and survival of these calves followed through the years of their lives. Other cohorts present in the population would be ignored. In contrast, a horizontal life table includes measurements about all individuals in the population at a particular time and several cohorts are included. All individuals within the various age classes are counted and the associated data summarized in a horizontal table. An important point to note here is that the results of cohort and horizontal life tables will not always be identical for the same population. They will be identical only if environmental conditions were sufficiently stable so that vital rates remained fairly independent of time, i.e. independent of the specific cohort(s) from which they were derived. In a composite life table, data are collected for several cohorts and combined. For example, a team of game managers might tag newborns during four consecutive calving seasons, follow the four cohorts through time, and combine the final results into one table.

5.1.2.1 Survival Schedules

Oh, Death, why canst thou sometimes be timely? (Melville, *Moby Dick* 1851)

Sometimes, life schedules quantify death only. Life insurance companies or some ecological risk assessors might correctly pay most attention to the likelihood of dying and consider natality as irrelevant. Such tabulations are called l_x schedules because, by convention, the symbol l_x designates the number of survivors in the age class, x. In some formulations, l_x is expressed as a proportion of the original number of newborns surviving to age x. In that form, it also estimates the probability of survival to age x.

From l_x schedules, simple estimates are made of the number of deaths ($d_x = l_x - l_{x+1}$), rate of mortality (q_x), and expected life time for an individual surviving to age x (e_x). Like l_x, if d_x is expressed as a proportion dying instead of actual number dying, d_x estimates the probability of dying in the interval x to $x + 1$. These estimates may be expressed as a simple quotient (e.g. $q_x = d_x/l_x$) or normalized to a specific number of individuals in the age class such as deaths per 1000 individuals (e.g. $1000\,q_x = 1000(d_x/l_x)$) (Deevey 1947).

The mean expected length of life beyond age x for an individual who survived to age x (e_x) can be estimated for any age class (x) by dividing the area under the survival curve after x by the number of individuals surviving to age x (Deevey 1947):

$$e_x = \frac{\int_x^\infty l_x \mathrm{d}x}{l_x} \tag{5.1}$$

With a basic l_x table, the e_x in equation (5.1) can be approximated with the l_x and L_x (number of living individuals between x and $x + 1$ in age):

$$L_x = \int_x^{x+1} l_x \mathrm{d}x \tag{5.2}$$

A simple linear approximation of L_x in equation (5.2) is $L_x = (l_x + l_{x+1})/2$. Obviously, the ∞ in the summations here and elsewhere become the age at the bottommost row of the completed life table. These L_x approximations are summed in the life table from the bottommost row up to and including the age of interest (x). The e_x value for an age class is then estimated by dividing this sum (T_x) by l_x, i.e. $e_x = T_x/l_x$. (The T_x is the total years lived by all individuals in the x age class.) The e_0 or expected life span for an individual at the beginning of the life table, i.e. a neonate, and its associated variance are estimated by Leslie *et al.* (1955) and described in detail by Krebs (1989).

A quick check of Section 3.1.3.1 (Accelerated Failure Time and Proportional Hazard Models) will show a striking similarity between those epidemiological methods for modeling mortality and these simple life table methods. In fact, the method just described is simply one method for summarizing survival information. Methods, models, and hypothesis tests described in Section 3.1.3.1 can be, and often are, applied in demography.

Box 5.1   Death, decline, and gamma rays

As the possibility of nuclear war emerged and our ignorance of its consequences became obvious, researchers in the 1950s and 1960s began to explore the ecological effects of intense irradiation. Ecological entities from individuals (e.g. Casarett 1968) to populations (e.g. Marshall 1962) to ecosystems (e.g. Woodwell 1962, 1963) were irradiated in innumerable studies to determine the consequences. One such study placed cultures of *Daphnia pulex* (50 individuals per culture) near a 5000 Curie cobalt (^{60}Co) source. The *Daphnia* experienced continuous gamma irradiation at dose rates of 0, 22.8, 47.9, 52.2, 67.5 and 75.9 Roentgens/h. Survival was monitored for 35 days and life schedules constructed for each irradiated population (Table 5.1). Instead of estimating a simple LD50 at a set time, Marshall (1962) used demographic methods to summarize the population consequences of irradiation. This allowed estimation of the change in average life expectancy as a consequence of dose rate (Figure 5.1). For the sake of brevity, calculations were done here by using weekly age classes, not daily age classes as done in the original publication. The original publication provides a more refined analysis of these data. Regardless, the decrease in average life expectancy for the different age classes was obvious. Note in Figure 5.1 that there is a suggestion of a hormetic effect at 22.8 Roentgens/h. (See Section 6.2 of Chapter 6 for discussion of hormesis.)

Obviously, survival functions and life expectancies provide valuable insights into population consequences and, when combined later with natality data (Example 5.2), of population fate under different intensities of irradiation.

Table 5.1. Survival rates (l_x as a proportion of the original population) for *Daphnia pulex* continuously irradiated with radiocobalt (modified from Table I in Marshall 1962)

Days (x)	Dose rate (Roentgens/h)					
	0	22.8	47.9	52.2	67.5	75.9
0	1.00	1.00	1.00	1.00	1.00	1.00
7	0.98	0.98	0.98	0.98	0.98	0.96
14	0.98	0.96	0.98	0.94	0.96	0.94
21	0.98	0.88	0.48	0.16	0.12	0.02
28	0.19	0.53	0.00	0.00	0.00	0.00
35	0.00	0.00	0.00	0.00	0.00	0.00

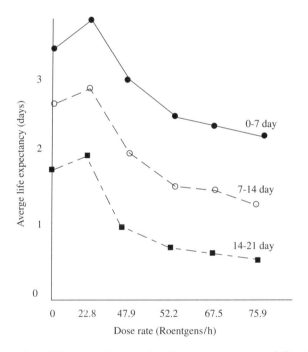

Fig. 5.1. Calculated life expectancies for three age classes of *Daphnia pulex* as a function of gamma irradiation dose rate

5.1.2.2 Mortality–natality tables

There is an appointed time for everything, and a time for every affair under the heavens. A time to be born, a time to die... (Ecclesiastes 3)

The inclusion of information on births (natality, m_x) in addition to mortality (l_x) allows expansion of this approach. The resulting schedules are called $l_x m_x$

tables. Often, $l_x m_x$ tables quantify information for females alone because the reproductive contribution of males to the next generation is much more difficult to estimate than that of females. For females, m_x is estimated as the average number of female offspring produced per female of age x. Several useful population qualities can be estimated after the age-specific birth rates (m_x) and l_x values are known. The expected number of female offspring produced in the life time of a female or net reproductive rate (R_0) is defined by equation (5.3) (Birch 1948):

$$R_0 = \int_0^\infty l_x m_x dx \qquad (5.3)$$

This ratio of female births in two successive generations is estimated as the sum of the products $l_x m_x$ for all age classes: $R_0 = \Sigma l_x m_x$. Knowing R_0, a mean generation time (T_c) can be calculated by dividing the sum of all the $x l_x m_x$ values by R_0. (The midpoint of interval x to $x + 1$ is used in the product, $x l_x m_x$. For example, $(0 + 1)/2$ or 0.5 would be used for x of the interval 0 to 1 year old.) It can also be estimated with equation (5.4); however, an estimate of the intrinsic rate of increase (r) would be needed:

$$T_c = \frac{\ln R_0}{r} \qquad (5.4)$$

The intrinsic rate of increase (r) could be grossly estimated with equation (5.5) which is a simple rearrangement of equation (5.4):

$$r = \frac{\ln R_0}{T_c} \qquad (5.5)$$

This gross estimate of r can then be used as an initial estimate in the Euler–Lotka equation (equation (5.6)) (Euler 1760; Lotka 1907) which becomes equation (5.7) for the approximate method applied to simple life tables (Birch 1948):

$$\int_0^\infty e^{-rx} l_x m_x dx = 1 \qquad (5.6)$$

$$\sum_{x=0}^{\omega} l_x m_x e^{-rx} = 1 \qquad (5.7)$$

where ω indicates the result for the bottommost row of the life table. The x, l_x, and m_x values, and the initial estimate of r from equation (5.5) are placed into equation (5.7), and the equation solved. Next, the value of r is changed slightly and the equation is solved again. This process is repeated with different estimates of r until a r is found for which the equality is 'close enough'. This final value of r is the best estimate from the life table. The assumptions here are that the population is increasing exponentially and the population is stable. However, Stearns (1992) indicates that this approach is robust to violations of the assumption of a stable age structure.

A stable population is one in which the distribution of individuals among the various age (or stage) classes remains constant. The structure of such a population is called its stable age structure. Any population with a constant r or λ will eventually take on a stable age structure: the distribution of individuals among the age classes will be a consequence of age-specific birth and death rates. The proportion of all individuals in age class x for a stable population (C_x) is defined by equation (5.8). (See Birch 1948; Stearns 1992; Newman 1995; or Caswell 1996 for more detail.)

$$C_x = \frac{\lambda^{-x} l_x}{\sum_{i=0}^{\omega} \lambda^{-i} l_i} \tag{5.8}$$

Remember from the previous chapter that $\lambda = e^r$.

Reproductive value (V_A) is a measure of the number of females that will be produced by a female of age A under the assumption of a stationary population. A stationary population is one in which simple replacement is occurring, i.e. $R_0 = 1$ or $r = 0$. Therefore, by definition, neonates will have a $V_A (= V_0)$ of 1 because each will just replace herself in a stationary population. Postreproductive females will have V_A values of 0. It follows that the V_A can be envisioned as the reproductive value for a specific class, x, divided by that of a neonate, i.e. $V_A = V_x/V_0$.

Age- or stage-specific reproductive values for a population are an extremely valuable set of metrics of the contribution of offspring to be expected from each age class to the next generation. The relative sizes of V_A values for the different age classes suggest the value of each age class in contributing new individuals to the next generation. It takes simultaneously into account the facts that a female has survived to age, x, and that she has an age-specific capacity to produce young. (See Wilson and Bossert (1971) or Stearns (1992) for a detailed description of V_A and detailed derivation of equations associated with V_A. Newman (1995) provides a detailed example of applying V_A to ecotoxicology.)

$$V_A = \sum_{x=A}^{\omega} \frac{l_x}{l_A} m_x \tag{5.9}$$

Goodman (1982, detailed in Stearns (1992)) provides equation (5.10), a modification of the Euler–Lotka equation, to describe V_A in an exponentially growing population. The lower contribution of offspring born later relative to the contribution of those born earlier is included in this equation (Wilson and Bossert 1971; Stearns 1992).

$$V_A = \frac{e^{r(A-1)}}{l_A} \sum_{x=A}^{\omega} e^{-rx} l_x m_x \tag{5.10}$$

This demographic metric provides valuable insights relevant to the weakest link incongruity. The reproductive value (V_A) suggests the loss in individuals that would otherwise come into the next generation if one individual of a certain age class were removed from the population. The most valuable individuals in this context are not always the young stages that are most sensitive to toxicant action. In general, one could argue that individuals just entering their reproductive stage might be more valuable as they usually have very high, reproductive values (Wilson and Bossert 1971). Regardless, conventional generalizations are insufficient that protection of the most sensitive stage based on most sensitive life stage testing will ensure a viable population. A thorough demographic analysis should be done in order to make any judgements about the population consequences of toxicant exposure.

There is also a definite linkage between this demographic concept of reproductive value and those described earlier for sustainable harvest. Due to aggregation of information, stimulation of harvest based solely on total numbers would be less effective than estimation based on a fuller knowledge of age- or size-specific harvests and reproductive values. Stock assessment models including size-specific harvesting gear have direct relevance to age-specific mortality in populations due to toxicant exposure.

Box 5.2 Death, decline, gamma rays, and birth

Marshall (1962) measured natality in addition to mortality for *Daphnia pulex* exposed to gamma radiation (Figure 5.1). Let's add these natality data (Table 5.2) to that already analyzed for mortality (Table 5.1). Again, data are pooled into weekly age classes.

Table 5.2. Natality (m_x) for *Daphnia pulex* continuously irradiated with radiocobalt (modified from Table II in Marshall 1962)

Day ($x - x + 1$)	Dose rate (Roentgens/h)					
	0	22.8	47.9	52.2	67.5	75.9
1-6	2.63	2.29	1.94	1.88	0.94	0.39
7-13	14.64	10.84	1.60	0.45	0.18	0.22
14-20	3.29	1.06	0.02			
21-27	0.35					
28-35	0.31					

The Euler–Lotka equation (equation (5.7)) was used to estimate the intrinsic rates of increase for the irradiated populations (Figure 5.2). Notice the general decrease in *r* until it drops below 0 at approximately 67.5 Roentgens/h. At that point, the population would slowly decrease to extinction. The stable population structures (Figure 5.3) showed a trend from a control population with many

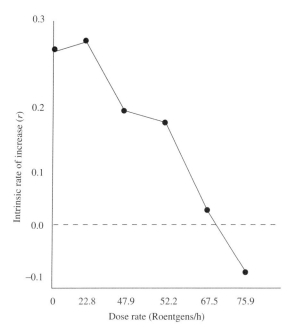

Fig. 5.2. Drop in intrinsic rate of increase (r) with dose rate for *Daphnia pulex* cultures

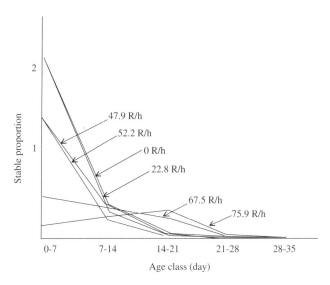

Fig. 5.3. Shift in stable population structure for *Daphnia pulex* cultures exposed to different dose rate of gamma radiation

young to highly dosed populations with proportionally few young and many old individuals. From the lowest to the highest dose, the generation times dropped rapidly from 13.6 to only 4.8–6.0 days.

Clearly, meaningful information relative to population changes and consequences were obtained from this simple demographic analysis. Irradiation reduced average life expectancy and generation time. Population growth rate decreased with dose until it fall below simple replacement at approximately 67.5 Roentgens/h. Populations receiving such doses would disappear after a few generations. The age structure of the populations shifted from control populations with many neonates to high dose populations with a preponderance of older individuals. These insights are much more meaningful than those provided by LD50 and NOEC data.

5.2 MATRIX FORMS OF DEMOGRAPHIC MODELS

To this point, discussion has been simplified by avoiding matrix algebra. However, the approach becomes much more powerful with matrix formulations for demographic qualities. Leslie (1945, 1948) produced a foundation approach to demographics based on simple matrix algebra. Consequently, any discussion of population demography neglecting matrix formulations is superficial. The rudimentary matrix operations needed to apply Leslie's approach and the fundamental approach of Leslie will be described in this section. The description of matrix mathematics in the next section come directly from Chapter 1 of Emlen (1984).

5.2.1 BASICS OF MATRIX CALCULATIONS

A matrix is simply a rectangular array of numbers or variables. Its size is usually designated by the number of rows (i) and columns (j), e.g. a 4×1 matrix or 4×4 matrix. A matrix composed of only one row is called a vector. A 1×1 matrix is a scalar, e.g. the number, 12, is a scalar:

$$\begin{bmatrix} 2 \\ 5 \\ 6 \\ 3 \end{bmatrix} = 4 \times 1 \text{ matrix} = \mathbf{a}$$

$$\begin{bmatrix} 12 & 5 & 17 & 3 \\ 23 & 0 & 12 & 10 \\ 5 & 5 & 5 & 3 \\ 12 & 7 & 13 & 5 \end{bmatrix} = 4 \times 4 \text{ matrix} = \mathbf{A}$$

Matrices are conventionally designated as boldfaced, capital letters (e.g. **A**), except vectors which are designated as boldface, small letters (e.g. **a** above). Scalars are written as small letters without boldfacing. A matrix can be denoted generally as $\mathbf{A} = \{a_{ij}\}$ where i designates row position and j designates column position. For example, element a_{13} in $\mathbf{A}$ above is 17.

We will need to do simple matrix multiplication in the demographic models that follow. Therefore, a quick review of matrix multiplication is presented here. Multiplication of a scalar by a matrix ($b \times \mathbf{A}$) is very straightforward. Each individual element of the matrix is simply multiplied by the scalar. Let b be a scalar with value 12 and $\mathbf{A}$ be a 2×2 matrix:

$$12 \times \mathbf{A} = 12 \begin{bmatrix} a_{11} & a_{12} \\ a_{21} & a_{22} \end{bmatrix} = \begin{bmatrix} 12a_{11} & 12a_{12} \\ 12a_{21} & 12a_{22} \end{bmatrix}$$

Multiplication of a matrix $\mathbf{A}$ by another matrix $\mathbf{B}$ is more tedious but no more difficult to grasp. The cross-products of the rows of $\mathbf{A}$ and columns of $\mathbf{B}$ are generated and summed as shown below. Let's use the $\mathbf{A}$ matrix (2×2) described immediately above and multiply it by another 2×2 matrix, $\mathbf{B}$:

$$\mathbf{A} \times \mathbf{B} = \begin{bmatrix} a_{11} & a_{12} \\ a_{21} & a_{22} \end{bmatrix} \times \begin{bmatrix} b_{11} & b_{12} \\ b_{21} & b_{22} \end{bmatrix} = \begin{bmatrix} a_{11}b_{11} + a_{12}b_{21} & a_{11}b_{12} + a_{12}b_{22} \\ a_{21}b_{11} + a_{22}b_{21} & a_{21}b_{12} + a_{22}b_{22} \end{bmatrix}$$

For example,

$$\mathbf{A} \times \mathbf{B} = \begin{bmatrix} 1 & 3 \\ 5 & 2 \end{bmatrix} \times \begin{bmatrix} 4 & 1 \\ 5 & 6 \end{bmatrix} = \begin{bmatrix} 4 + 15 & 1 + 18 \\ 20 + 10 & 5 + 12 \end{bmatrix} = \begin{bmatrix} 19 & 19 \\ 30 & 17 \end{bmatrix}$$

Multiplication of a matrix ($\mathbf{A}$) and a vector ($\mathbf{b}$) is done in the same way:

$$\mathbf{A} \times \mathbf{b} = \begin{bmatrix} a_{11} & a_{12} \\ a_{21} & a_{22} \end{bmatrix} \times \begin{bmatrix} b_{11} \\ b_{21} \end{bmatrix} = \begin{bmatrix} a_{11}b_{11} + a_{12}b_{21} \\ a_{21}b_{11} + a_{22}b_{21} \end{bmatrix}$$

We can demonstrate this multiplication by modifying the above example:

$$\mathbf{A} \times \mathbf{b} = \begin{bmatrix} 1 & 3 \\ 5 & 2 \end{bmatrix} \times \begin{bmatrix} 4 \\ 5 \end{bmatrix} = \begin{bmatrix} 4 + 15 \\ 20 + 10 \end{bmatrix} = \begin{bmatrix} 19 \\ 30 \end{bmatrix}$$

5.2.2 THE LESLIE MATRIX APPROACH

The reason that we spent a moment reviewing matrix multiplication is that, more than half a century ago, Leslie (1945, 1948) took the natality and mortality rates from life tables and expressed them using simple matrix algebra. He placed the probability (P_x) of a female alive at time period x to $x + 1$ surviving during period $x + 1$ to $x + 2$ in the subdiagonal of a matrix and the numbers of daughters (F_x) born in time t to $t + 1$ per female of age x to $x + 1$ in the top row of a square

$(\omega \times \omega)$ matrix (**L**). The remaining matrix elements were 0's:

$$
\mathbf{L} =
\begin{bmatrix}
0 & F_1 & F_2 & F_3 & \dots & F_\omega \\
P_0 & 0 & 0 & 0 & \dots & 0 \\
0 & P_1 & 0 & 0 & \dots & 0 \\
0 & 0 & P_2 & 0 & \dots & 0 \\
\dots & \dots & \dots & \dots & \dots & \dots \\
0 & 0 & 0 & 0 & P_{\omega-1} & 0
\end{bmatrix}
$$

The conditions for this Leslie matrix being valid were $0 < P_x < 1$ and $F_x \geq 0$. The ratio of the two sexes may be included in the matrix by multiplying the F_x values calculated by combining both sexes by the sex ratio, f_x, and using that product instead of the F_x values. Among the many convenient aspects of this matrix formulation of demographic vital rates, this matrix (**L**) can be multiplied by a vector ($\mathbf{n}_t$) of the number of individuals at the various x ages to predict the number of individuals in each age class at some time in the future, e.g. the *Daphnia* populations described in Tables 5.1 and 5.2:

$$
\mathbf{L} \times \mathbf{n} =
\begin{bmatrix}
F_0 & F_1 & F_2 & F_3 & \dots & F_\omega \\
P_0 & 0 & 0 & 0 & \dots & 0 \\
0 & P_1 & 0 & 0 & \dots & 0 \\
0 & 0 & P_2 & 0 & \dots & 0 \\
\dots & \dots & \dots & \dots & \dots & \dots \\
0 & 0 & 0 & 0 & P_\omega - 1 & 0
\end{bmatrix}
\times
\begin{bmatrix}
n_{0,t} \\ n_{1,t} \\ n_{2,t} \\ n_{3,t} \\ \dots \\ n_{\omega,t}
\end{bmatrix}
=
\begin{bmatrix}
n_{0,t+1} \\ n_{1,t+1} \\ n_{2,t+1} \\ n_{3,t+1} \\ \dots \\ n_{\omega,t+1}
\end{bmatrix}
$$

The Leslie matrix can be multiplied by this new vector of age class sizes for $t + 1$ to project the population characteristics at time $t + 2$. The process can be repeated for $t + 3$ and so on through many time steps. Emlen (1984) provides the following simple example of this process. Let the initial population be composed of 200 neonates with the population demographics summarized by the Leslie matrix, **L**

$$
\mathbf{n_0} =
\begin{bmatrix}
200 \\ 0 \\ 0
\end{bmatrix}
$$

The vector of age-class sizes after one time step, $\mathbf{n}_1$ is equal to $\mathbf{L} \times \mathbf{n}_0$:

$$
\mathbf{n_1} = \mathbf{L} \times \mathbf{n_0} =
\begin{bmatrix}
0 & 1 & 4 \\
0.5 & 0 & 0 \\
0 & 0.25 & 0
\end{bmatrix}
\times
\begin{bmatrix}
200 \\ 0 \\ 0
\end{bmatrix}
=
\begin{bmatrix}
0 \\ 100 \\ 0
\end{bmatrix}
$$

Obviously from the F_0 element of **L**, the neonates do not reproduce during their first x to $x + 1$ time of life so the number of newborns at time step 1 is 0. Half of the yearlings die in x to $x + 1$ so the size of this cohort drops from the original 200 to 100. And with a second time step,

$$
\mathbf{n_2} = \mathbf{L} \times \mathbf{n_1} =
\begin{bmatrix}
0 & 1 & 4 \\
0.5 & 0 & 0 \\
0 & 0.25 & 0
\end{bmatrix}
\times
\begin{bmatrix}
0 \\ 100 \\ 0
\end{bmatrix}
=
\begin{bmatrix}
100 \\ 0 \\ 25
\end{bmatrix}
$$

Now the 100 individuals have moved into a reproductive stage of their lives, resulting in $100(= 100 \times 1)$ newborns. Because the survival of the original cohort was only expected to be 0.25 for the next step, only 100×0.25 or 25 remain. Additional iterations could be carried out to track the population further through time but the method has been demonstrated sufficiently with these few steps.

Other calculations can be performed with this approach and only a few are presented here. As examples, the right and left eigenvectors of the Leslie matrix define the stable age structure and age-specific reproductive values for the population, respectively. Migration into the population each time step can be included as $\mathbf{n}_{t+1} = \mathbf{Ln}_t + \mathbf{m}_t$ where $\mathbf{m}_t$ is a vector containing the number of migrants of the various age classes appearing during the time step. Growth can be included in the matrix. The reader is directed to Leslie (1945, 1948) or Caswell (1989, 1996) for further details.

5.2.3 STOCHASTIC MODELS

The certainty of death is attended with uncertainties in time, manner, places. (Thomas Browne cited in Deevey 1947)

If vital rates were defined as variable, the deterministic matrix approach just described could be expanded to a stochastic one. For example, the replicate *Daphnia* cultures for the six gamma irradiation treatments could have been used to define the variance to be anticipated in vital rates. At each time step, the vital rates are drawn randomly from distributions and applied as described above. The population size and structure would then be characterized by a stochastic trajectory through time. If this process was repeated many times as done with Monte Carlo simulation, a family of possible outcomes could be generated. The probability of local extinction or of falling below a certain population size (M) could be estimated from the outcomes of such simulations. For example, 234 of 1000 simulations of a toxicant-exposed population might have produced populations that fell to size 0, suggesting that nearly one quarter of populations are predicted to go locally extinct under those exposure conditions. Because the Allee effect suggests that some populations might have minimal sizes (M) above 0 that must be maintained in order to remain viable, some other threshold population size might be used instead of 0. The RAMAS program (Ferson and Akçakaya 1990) performs the calculations described here for deterministic and stochastic models. This affords the expression of population change due to toxicant exposure as a true risk. (A statement of risk must include the probability of an adverse effect and the magnitude of the effect.) For example, a specific exposure may result in a 1 in 10 chance of the population size dropping by 50% during the 10 years that the toxicant remains above a certain threshold concentration in the species' habitat. Such models may also be developed in a metapopulation framework.

5.3 SUMMARY

This chapter demonstrates the basics of demography and their utility in population ecotoxicology. For example, the analysis of *Daphnia pulex* population response to gamma irradiation described here is much more meaningful than the conventional ecotoxicology approach in which a LC50 for lethality and NOEC for reproductive effects are generated. With the demographic methods, a clear consequence is indicated by the r falling below 0 at a dose rate of approximately 67.5 Roentgens/h. Even more useful information would be obtained with the inclusion of stochastic considerations. In contrast, the gross metrics of LC50 or NOEC would force the application of large uncertainty factors in order to accommodate the associated inaccuracy of these metrics of effect. Fortunately, more and more demographic analyses are being done for the effects of pollutants. Sibly (1996) provides a literature search of such studies, indicating the value of the approach. Hopefully, the trend toward such population methods will continue during the next decade.

5.3.1 SUMMARY OF FOUNDATION CONCEPTS AND PARADIGMS

- Populations have structure relative to age and sex, and this structure can be influenced by toxicant exposure.

- Toxicant exposure can modify vital rates and, consequently, population qualities and viability.

- Conventional life table and matrix methods allow description and quantitative prediction of population qualities.

- Results of life table analyses complement those described in Chapter 3 for survival analysis.

- Life table analysis is possible for groups of individuals exposed in laboratory toxicity tests.

- Metrics from demographic analysis are useful for defining population status under the influence of toxicant exposure.

- Demographic qualities of some species make them more or less susceptible to toxicant effects and, consequently, metrics derived for effects to individuals only are poor predictors of population effects to some species.

- Demographic metrics are compatible with wildlife management, fisheries stock management, and conservation biology metrics of population status.

- Potential measures of effect include r, λ, V_A, stable population structure, and probability of local extinction.

- Toxicants can influence migration into and out of populations by modifying mechanisms such as avoidance, drift, and territoriality.

REFERENCES

Bechmann RK (1994). Use of life tables and LC50 tests to evaluate chronic and acute toxicity effects of copper on the marine copepod *Tisbe furcata* (Baird). *Environ Toxicol Chem* **13**: 1509–1517.

Birch LC (1948). The intrinsic rate of natural increase in an insect population. *J Animal Ecol* **17**: 15–26.

Casarett A (1968). *Radiation Biology*. Prentice Hall, Englewood Cliffs, NJ.

Caswell H (1989). *Matrix Population Models: Construction, Analysis, and Interpretation*. Sinauer Associates, Inc., Sunderland, MA.

Caswell H (1996). Demography meets ecotoxicology: untangling the population level effects of toxic substances. In *ecotoxicology. A Hierarchical Treatment*, ed. by MC Newman and CH. Jagoe, pp. 255–292. CRC/Lewis Press, Boca Raton, FL.

Daniels RE and Allan JD (1981). Life table evaluation of chronic exposure to a pesticide. *Can J Fish Aquat Sci* **38**: 485–494.

Day K and Kaushik NK (1987). An assessment of the chronic toxicity of the synthetic pyrethroid, Fenvalerate, to *Daphnia galeata mendotae*, using life tables. *Environ Toxicol* **44**: 13–26.

Deevey Jr ES (1947). Life tables for natural populations of animals. *Q Rev Biol* **22**: 283–314.

Emlen JM (1984). *Population Biology. The Coevolution of Population Dynamics and Behavior*. Macmillan, New York.

Euler L (1760). Recherches générales sur la mortalité: la multiplication du benre humain. *Mem Acad Sci, Berlin* **16**: 144–164.

Ferson S and Akçakaya HR (1990). *Modeling Fluctuations in Age-structured Populations. RAMAS/age User Manual*. Applied Biomathematics, Setauket, NY.

Goodman D (1982). Optimal life histories, optimal notation, and the value of reproductive value. *Am Nat* **119**: 803–823.

Kammenga JE, Busschers M, Van Straalen NM, Jepson PC, and Baker J (1996). Stress induced fitness is not determined by the most sensitive life-cycle trait. *Funct Ecol* **10**: 106–111.

Koivisto S and Ketola M (1995). Effects of copper on life-history traits of *Daphnia pulex* and *Bosmina longirostris*. *Aquat Toxicol* **32**: 255–269.

Krebs CJ (1989). *Ecological Methodology*. HarperCollins, New York.

Leslie, PH (1945). On the use of matrices in certain population mathematics. *Biometrika* **33**: 183–212.

Leslie PH (1948). Some further notes on the use of matrices in population mathematics. *Biometrika* **35**: 213–245.

Leslie PH, Tener JS, Vizoso M and Chitty H (1955). The longevity and fertility of the Orkney vole, *Microtus orcadensis*, as observed in the laboratory. *Proc Zool Soc London* **125**: 115–125.

Lotka AJ (1907). Studies on the mode of growth of material aggregates. *Am J Sci* **24**: 199–216.

Marshall JS (1962). The effects of continuous gamma radiation on the intrinsic rate of natural increase of *Daphnia pulex*. *Ecology* **43**: 598–607.

Martinez-Jerónimo F, Villaseñor R, Espinosa F and Rios G (1993). Use of life-tables and application factors for evaluating chronic toxicity of Kraft mill wastes on *Daphnia magna*. *Bull Environ Contam Toxicol* **50**: 377–384.

Münzinger A and Guarducci M.-L (1988). The effect of low zinc concentrations on some demographic parameters of *Biomphalaria glabrata* (Say), mollusca: gastropoda. *Aquat Toxicol* **12**: 51–61.

Munns Jr WR, Black DE, Gleason TR, Salomon K, Bengtson D and Gutjanr-Gobell R (1997). Evaluation of the effects of dioxin and PCBs on *Fundulus heteroclitus* populations using a modeling approach. *Environ Toxicol Chem* **16**: 1074–1081.

Newman MC (1995). *Quantitative Methods in Aquatic Ecotoxicology*. CRC/Lewis Press, Boca Raton, FL.

Newman MC (1998). Fundamentals of Ecotoxicology. Ann Arbor Press, Chelsea, MI.

Pesch CE, Munns Jr WR and Gutjahr-Gobell R (1991). Effects of a contaminated sediment on life history traits and population growth rate of *Neanthes arenaceodentata* (Polychaeta: Nereidae) in the laboratory. *Environ Toxicol Chem* **10**: 805–815.

Petersen Jr RC and Petersen LB-M (1988). Compensatory mortality in aquatic populations: its importance for interpretation of toxicant effects. *Ambio* **17**: 381–386.

Sibly RM (1996). Effects of pollutants on individual life histories and population growth rates. In *Ecotoxicology. A Hierarchical Treatment* ed. by MC Newman and CH Jagoe, pp. 197–223. CRC/Lewis Press, Boca Raton, FL.

Stearns SC (1992). *The Evolution of Life Histories*. Oxford University Press, Oxford.

Wilson EO and Bossert WH (1971). *A Primer of Population Biology*. Sinauer Associates, Inc., Sunderland, MA.

Woodwell GM (1962). Effects of ionizing radiation on terrestrial ecosystems. *Science* **138**: 572–577.

Woodwell GM (1963). The ecological effects of radiation. *Sci Am* **208**: 2–11.

6 The Phenotype in Exposed Populations

...it would be well if men's minds were accustomed to, and that early, that they might not erect their opinions upon one single view, when so many other are requisite to make up the account, and must come into the reckoning before a man can form a right judgement. (Locke 1706)

6.1 OVERVIEW

6.1.1 THE PHENOTYPE VANTAGE

The need for theories linking physiological and population effects is particularly strong in ecotoxicology: toxic substances affect the physiological behavior of individuals but the environmental problems occur at the population and ecosystem level. (Kooijman, Van der Hoeven and Van der Werf 1989)

...physiological response to toxicants at an individual level can be related rigorously to predict population dynamics responses. The link can be achieved straightforwardly provided functional relationships between various physiological responses and survivorship, fecundity and developmental rates [i.e. vital rates] *can be established.* (Calow and Sibly 1990)

The translation from a pollutant's effects on individuals to its effects on the population can be accomplished using life-history analysis to calculate the effect on the population's growth rate. (Sibly 1996)

Conventional descriptions of contaminant effects to populations give short shrift to the root of effects, i.e. toxicant-induced, phenotypic changes to life history traits. Notable exceptions include the work of McFarlane and Franzin (1978) and Maltby (1991) with aquatic organisms and Kammenga *et al.* (1996) with soil nematodes. Ecotoxicologists often consider the phenotype solely in the context of biochemical, physiological, toxicokinetic, and toxicological characteristics of individuals. Only vague speculation is applied to linking phenotypic traits to population consequences. This chapter attempts to move outside of that context to develop a vantage of population effects emerging from toxicant-induced changes to phenotypes.

Phenotypic variations in rates of growth and development, onset and rate of reproduction, and rate of mortality will be described and linked to emergent population consequences. Therefore, discussion will move between the individual and population context to achieve a more inclusive whole. The overriding themes are the following: (1) translation of phenotypic differences in life history traits of individuals into population consequences, (2) change in Darwinian fitness associated with these life history phenotypes, and (3) potential for adaptation and microevolution. These themes are based on the causal sequence that phenotypic variation in life history traits of exposed individuals produce changes in population vital rates. Shifts in population vital rates can give rise to diminished population viability, demographic change, or life history adaptation and microevolution.

The influence of toxicants on the capacity within a population to produce a consistent phenotype (i.e. developmental stability) will be described at the end of the chapter. Deviations from perfect developmental stability will be discussed as population-level indicators of contaminant effect.

6.1.2 AN EXTREME CASE EXAMPLE

Species populations differ relative to how life history traits expressed under various conditions will influence population qualities. This can be made obvious by quickly reviewing the classic r- (opportunistic) and k- (equilibrial) selection context for population strategy (Table 6.1). Species at the two extremes of this scheme respond differently to stressors, and as a consequence, species populations at the ends of this continuum often have different fates under identical exposure scenarios. Acute exposure that eliminates nearly all individuals from a habitat might have a trivial consequence to the persistence of an r-selected species that will quickly repopulate the area via migration and rapid reproduction. The opportunistic r-strategist has life history traits allowing it to bounce back and quickly reestablish itself after an unpredictable stress has occurred. With the r-selected species' tendency toward semelparity (an individual reproduces in a single pulse during its lifetime, e.g. an annual plant), the rate of recolonization might be quite stochastic and season dependent. In contrast, a K-selected species might take much longer to recover due to its lower rate of reproduction. Although it is risky to predict too far up the ecological hierarchy from individual life history traits, the general community-level consequence is that toxicant-exposed community composition shifts away from K-strategists in favor of r-strategists (May 1976; Odum 1985). Relationships have also been suggested specifically between tolerance to toxicants and the r- and K-strategies of fish (Neuhold 1987) and nematodes (Bongers and Ferris 1999). A soil nematode community metric of toxicant effect is based on the shift in community composition to favor r-strategists (Bongers 1990; Bongers and Ferris 1999). For both types of strategists, the range of phenotypes and possible changes in life history-related phenotypes at exposure will dictate short- and long term consequences to populations and communities.

The r- and K-strategist scheme is a convenient oversimplification; however, its application here provides a valid extreme-case illustration for considering life history traits when predicting population consequences. In reality, most species fit along a continuum of life history strategies ranging from pure r- to pure

Table 6.1. Themes in populations dominated by r- or K-selection strategies (modified from Neuhold 1987 and May 1976)

Characteristic	r-strategy	K-strategy
Strategy	Opportunistic, emphasis on producing large numbers of offspring quickly	Efficient interspecific competitor for resources; emphasis on producing few, high-quality offspring
Habitat	Temporary or variable, unpredictable, often 'ecological vacuums' not requiring efficient competition (May 1976)	Stable and predictable
Mortality	High; migration may be important, Deevey Type I mortality curve (Deevey 1947)	Returns to K after perturbation; Deevey Type II or III mortality curve (Deevey 1947)
Strategy favors	Rapid development to sexual maturity High r, 'boom–bust' population dynamics Low investment in individual offspring Small body size Short lifespan and generation time Semelparity (single reproductive event/individual)	Slow development to sexual maturity Efficient competitor in community High investment in individual offspring Large body size Long lifespan and generation time Iteroparity (several reproductive events/individual)

K-strategists. Some species tend toward one strategy at one stage of their life cycle (e.g. larval amphibians living in temporary ponds) and a second strategy at another stage (e.g. terrestrial adult amphibians). Regardless, the suite of life history traits that combine to create these strategies is subject to natural selection. Some traits can change as the environment changes so the capacity of the phenotype to change in response to environmental cues is also subject to natural selection.

Many changes in phenotype in response to toxicant exposure can be readily associated with enhancement of individual fitness, e.g. induction of a detoxification mechanism enhances survival. But all crucial changes are not so obvious (e.g. Box 6.1). Less obvious are increases in fitness due to shifts in suites of individual life history characteristics. Our discussion of such changes, beginning here with the extremes of r- and K-strategists under toxicant stress, will now be expanded to include more subtle, but equally important, life history shifts.

Long-term consequences of the capacity to modify life history traits are also important to understanding this facet of population ecotoxicology. Potential for rapid evolution of life history traits in response to toxicant exposure exists. The rate of evolution of life history traits in response to non-toxicant environmental factors can be very rapid (Svensson 1997) and similar rates might be expected for toxicant-related changes.

Box 6.1 The weakest link incongruity: compensatory mortality in caddisfly populations

As mentioned in previous chapters, toxicity testing protocols supporting environmental regulation focus on the most sensitive stage of the life history. A critical life stage test, often an early life stage test, is performed to estimate a toxicant concentration with no or negligible effect (maximum acceptable toxicant concentration or MATC). Although the associated logic is sound if the focus remains on protecting individuals, an incongruity (weakest link incongruity (Newman 1998)) emerges when such results are used to imply a concentration below which the population is protected. The most toxicant-sensitive stage of an individual's life may or may not be the most critical stage in determining the demographic consequences of exposure. Along with many other factors, compensatory mortality (illustrated below) confounds such predictions of population fate.

In a study of pulp mill contaminants, Petersen and Petersen (1988) exposed various larval stages of the net-spinning hydropsychid caddisfly, *Hydrophsyche siltalai*, to 4,5,6-trichloroguaiacol. Because significant density-dependent mortality occurs at early stages (≤ 9 days) of this insect's life, Petersen and Petersen hypothesized that a clear concentration–response relationship might be difficult to generate for this putatively most sensitive stage. Reduced larval densities in the highest concentration treatments due to toxicity-induced mortality would result in lower levels of the natural, density-dependent mortality in the ≤ 9-day larvae. Rates of density-dependent mortality might be significantly different in low and high concentration treatments. A nonadditive combination of natural, density-dependent mortality and density-independent, toxicant-induced mortality would occur in the test chambers. Changes in natural, density-dependent mortality could compensate for changes in toxicant-related mortality. The relationship between toxicant concentration and mortality could be obscured as a consequence.

Older stages of this caddisfly exhibit much lower levels of natural, density-dependent mortality. Petersen and Petersen showed that these older larval stages have a clearer relationship between concentration and lethal effect. Figure 6.1 demonstrates the confounding effect of density-dependent, natural mortality for early stages (≤ 9 days of age), but not for older larvae.

The density dependence of early life stage mortality for this species must be considered in identifying the 'most sensitive life stage' for making accurate predictions of toxicant effects *to populations*. This potential for compensatory mortality is relevant to many other species, including many fishes (Petersen and Petersen 1988).

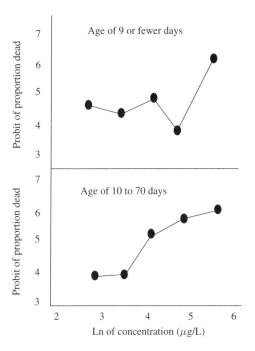

Fig. 6.1. Density-dependent, natural mortality can obscure the concentration–effect relationship for caddisfly larvae exposed to 4,5,6-trichloroguaiacol. There was no discernible relationship for larvae ≤9 days old, an age class with high levels of natural, density-dependent death. Note the high mortality in all treatments. (Probit values of 4 and 5 correspond to 16 and 50% mortality, respectively.) There was a clear relationship between mortality and toxicant concentration of older larvae (>9 to 70 days old). (Modified from Figure 4A&B of Petersen and Petersen 1988)

6.2 TOXICANTS AND THE PRINCIPLE OF ALLOCATION (CONCEPT OF STRATEGY)

Organisms have a finite amount of energy available to fulfill their diverse life functions and they must follow some basic rules when using this energy. For example, Selye (1956, 1973) described the general adaptation syndrome (GAS) for an individual's response to stress. The central theme of the GAS is that mechanisms are induced in response to stressors to resist change to normal homeostasis of the individual. Short-term, but energetically demanding, responses, such as a rapid increase in pulse and blood pressure, occur immediately after stress. Lower cost, more long-term, mechanisms emerge (e.g. enlargement of the adrenal cortex) if stress continues. If the stress intensity and duration exceeds the individual's finite energetic resources, the organism goes into an exhaustion phase and eventually dies.

Selye formulated this stress theory based on the response of wounded soldiers to physical stress. Consequently, the Selyean stress theory describes energy-demand compensating changes within individuals without consideration of functions other than survival.

Expanding the GAS to a life cycle context involving functions other than survival, the K-rule ('Kappa-rule') specifies that energy be meted out in a particular way among somatic maintenance, growth, development, and reproduction (Figure 6.2, top). A portion (K) is used for maintenance and growth with any remaining ($1-K$) being allocated to reproduction and/or development (Kooijman 1993). Maintenance is given top priority with growth being the next priority. Any energy for development is first spent to maintain a basal rate of maturation with an increase from this basal rate only if additional energy is available. Such straightforward rules for energy allocation have manifestations at the level of the population. In the remainder of this section and Section 6.2.3, more involved, epiphenomenal rules of energy utilization will be explored.

Extending the basic K-rule to the principle of allocation (concept of strategy) (Levins 1968), an individual with a specific genetic make-up and living in a particular environment must allocate energy resources so as to maximize its Darwinian fitness (Figure 6.2, bottom). The principal of allocation stipulates that there exists a trade-off for each allocation. Energy spent on one function, process, or structure cannot be used for another. If *Daphnia pulex* puts resources into growing spines that reduce predation risk (Kreuger and Dodson 1981), these resources are not available for egg production. Similarly, energy spent by an exposed individual to produce a detoxification enzyme or to replace toxicant-damaged proteins is not available for somatic growth or reproduction. (Protein turn over and synthesis costs in excess of 15% of basal metabolism in mammals; so, the additional cost of toxicant-related protein replacement or production of detoxification proteins can be high (Sibly and Calow 1989).) As evidence of such a trade-off, Adams *et al.* (1992) noted that redbreast sunfish (*Lepomis auritus*) exposed to a mixture of contaminants in East Fork Poplar Creek (Oak Ridge, Tennessee) displayed increased detoxification enzyme levels but low lipid levels, decreased growth rate, and depressed reproduction.

A best strategy exists for doling out resources and the capacity of individuals to modify allocation toward optimal allocation is subject to natural selection. Traits most often considered in optimality studies include metabolic maintenance, somatic growth, reproduction, survival (including longevity), and foraging (Stearns 1992; Atchison, Sandheinrich and Bryan 1996). Obviously, phylogenetic differences dictate limits to the possible range of traits a species can display and,

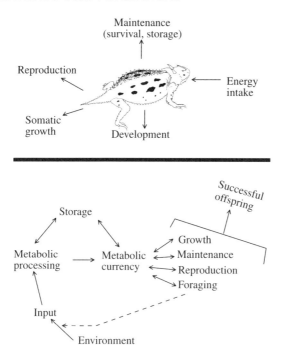

Fig. 6.2. The allocation of energy resources among essential functions of an individual. Organisms must optimize the environment-specific trade-off in resource allocation into life history components in order to achieve the highest Darwinian fitness. Energy spent on maintenance can include that associated with detoxification mechanisms, toxicant-induced changes in structures, active elimination of toxicants and metabolites, repair of damage, and other mechanisms associated with tolerance enhancement. (Modified from Figure 1 in Watt 1986)

bounded by these constraints, phenotypic variations exist within a species. For example, phylogenetically correlated differences in species groupings such as endotherm versus ectotherm or environmental conformer versus regulator bring about differences in basic allocation strategies and define their limits.

The principle of allocation is relevant to the outwardly enigmatic phenomenon of hormesis. Hormesis, the stimulatory effect exhibited with exposure to low, subinhibitory levels of some toxicants, is often observed for life-history traits such as somatic growth, reproduction, and survival (see Figure 5.1). For example, application of low doses of the growth retardant, phosfon, to the mint, *Mentha piperita*, actually stimulates growth (Calabrese, McCarthy and Kenyon 1987). Hormesis is noted occasionally for population growth which, in this chapter, is seen as a consequence emerging from changes in individual life-history traits.

Hormesis is often presented in ecotoxicology as an exceptional and counter-intuitive phenomenon — a peculiarity. Enhanced DNA repair due to radiation at low levels was recently described by Sagan (1989) as a 'surprising possibility'. Earlier, Sagan (1987) explained that '...frequent reports in the literature of "anomalies" at low doses...have been referred to as "hormetic" effects'. Oddly, a century before these statements were made, the principle of hormesis was sufficiently well known to be identified as the Arndt-Schulz Law, Hueppe's Rule, Sufficient Challenge, and hormoligosis (Stebbing 1982; Calabrese McCarthy and Kenyon 1987).

Although difficult to explain within traditional ecotoxicological paradigms, hormesis is one obvious manifestation of the principal of allocation. Reallocation of energy among somatic growth, reproduction, and maintenance (survival) will vary among some, but not necessarily all, species-toxicant combinations. An increase in growth at low concentrations might be expected if energy is shifted toward somatic maintenance and away from reproduction. Hormesis is a predictable outcome of the reallocation of energy resources as environmental conditions shift. It is not surprising that the magnitude of effect does not always conform to a monotonic trend with toxicant concentration. Compensatory reallocation of resources combines in a complex way with adverse toxic effects occurring at the various exposure levels. Depending on the capacity of the individual to reallocate resources and its particular strategy, hormesis could be one predictable outcome of low level exposure. Hormesis appears enigmatic only when one life history trait is studied in isolation from others.

6.2.1 PHENOTYPIC PLASTICITY AND NORMS OF REACTION

Reaction norms transform environmental variation into phenotypic variation...Reaction norms can be either inflexible, in which a characteristic once determined is never changed later in the organism's life, or they can be flexible, in which a characteristic can be altered more than once in the development of the same individual. (Stearns 1989)

The phenotype is a consequence of genetic (G) and environmental (E) factors, and the interaction between these factors (G × E). An individual has the potential to express a range of phenotypes depending on its environmental setting and genetic make-up. The reaction norm concept (Woltereck 1909) is used to describe this phenotypic plasticity relative to life history traits and is often applied to study optimization of Darwinian fitness. (The opposite of phenotypic plasticity is environmental canalization in which a consistent phenotype is produced regardless of environmental conditions (Stearns 1989).) Typically, reaction norms are represented as shown in Figure 6.3. Under a range of intensities of some environmental quality (e.g, temperature, moisture, or toxicant concentration), the genetic characteristics of the individual can translate into one of a range of phenotypes (Figure 6.3, top). The reaction norm might be linear (Figure 6.3, top) or curvilinear (Figure 6.3, bottom), and genotypes within a population can have distinct reaction norms (Genotypes A, B, and C in Figure 6.3, bottom). A G × E interaction is evident when reaction norms for different genotypes (or genetic lineages)

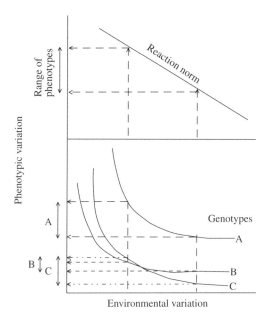

Fig. 6.3. The reaction norm shows the translation of genotype into a range of phenotypes as a consequence of environmental variation. In the top panel (modified from Stearns 1989), variation in the environment (*x* axis) results in variation in expressed phenotype (*y* axis) for a particular genotype. The relationship is linear in this example. In the bottom panel, reaction norms for several genotypes are shown as curvilinear. A genetic × environmental interaction exists if reaction norms for different genotypes cross one another. Note the distinct ranges of potential phenotypes for the three genotypes (double-headed arrows on *y* axis of bottom panel)

cross as shown for Genotypes B and C in the bottom panel of Figure 6.3. The reaction norm and conceptually similar approaches have been applied to relative fitnesses of metal tolerant and intolerant plants under a range of metal exposures (Hickey and McNeilly 1975), populations of metal-exposed midges (Posthuma, van Kleunen and Admiraal 1995), *Drosophila melanogaster* experiencing diverse environmental stresses (Clark 1997), and responses of different populations of zooplankton to metal contamination (Forbes *et al.* 1999).

Box 6.2 Applying reaction norms to mercury-exposed mosquitofish

Mulvey *et al.* (1995) applied the reaction norm approach to assess the influence of mosquitofish (*Gambusia holbrooki*) genotype on mercury sensitivity. Four mesocosms containing 985 mosquitofish each were split into two groups; a pair of untreated mesocosms and a pair of mesocosms spiked weekly to a water concentration of 18 µg/L of mercury. A third pair of mesocosms had also been spiked to 42 µg/L but no mosquitofish in this treatment survived to the end of the experiment. After 111 days, fish were harvested and measurements made of a variety of genetic and life history traits. Female life history traits measured for the different genotypes included number of late stage embryos carried by a gravid female, percentage of adult females that were gravid, and fish size (standard length). The fish populations in the control mesocosms doubled in number and those in the 18 µg/L treatment dropped approximately 25% by the end of the experiment.

Putative genotypes for the glycolytic enzyme, glucosephosphate isomerase-2 (*Gpi-2*), were determined by starch gel electrophoresis. Three alleles (38, 66, and the 100 common allele) were scored but, because of the low frequency of some genotypes in some mesocosms, the uncommon genotypes (38 and 66) were pooled and designated as '+' to produce three possible genotypes of 100/100, 100/+, and +/+. Responses of females of these genotypic designations were plotted for the two treatments (Figure 6.4).

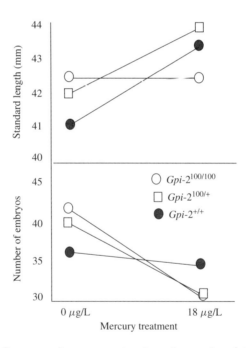

Fig. 6.4. The influence of mercury treatment on size (standard length) and fecundity (number of late stage embryos/gravid female) of female mosquitofish. Modified from Figure 3 in Mulvey *et al.* (1995)

Female standard length remained relatively unaffected by mercury treatment for the *Gpi-2*[100/100] homozygotes but was greater for the *Gpi-2*[100/+]

and $Gpi\text{-}2^{+/+}$ genotypes. Note that crossing of the reaction norms for the different genotypes indicates a genetic $\times$ environment (G $\times$ E) interaction: the different genotypes responded differently to the presence of mercury in the environment. Similarly, the number of late stage embryos carried by the females of the $Gpi\text{-}2^{+/+}$ genotype changed little with mercury additions. In contrast, the other genotypes ($Gpi\text{-}2^{100/100}$ and $Gpi\text{-}2^{100/+}$) had significantly fewer late stage embryos. Again, there was a clear G $\times$ E interaction. The genotypes responded differently to mercury exposure relative to these important life history traits, suggesting the potential for selection at the $Gpi\text{-}2$ locus (or a closely linked locus) during multiple generations of mercury exposure. (See Tatara, Mulvey and Newman (1999) for a description of the multiple generation consequences to mosquitofish in these mesocosms.)

Although not shown in Figure 6.4, there were other differences in reproduction among exposed genotypes. The percentage of adult females that were gravid was similar (*circa* 70%) for the three genotypes in the control mesocosms. The percentages of gravid females of the $Gpi\text{-}2^{100/+}$ and $Gpi\text{-}2^{+/+}$ genotypes from the mercury-treated mesocosm were also approximately 70%; only 43% of the $Gpi\text{-}2^{100/100}$ females in the mercury-treated mesocosm were gravid. If plotted as a reaction norm, a G $\times$ E interaction would be clear for the $Gpi\text{-}2^{100/100}$ genotype; again, suggesting a shift away from resource allocation to reproduction by the $Gpi\text{-}2^{100/100}$ homozygote during mercury exposure.

These differences in fish size (standard length), fecundity (number of late stage embryos), and percentage gravid females can be viewed from the vantage of energy trade-offs. For all genotypes, fish size increased and investment in young (late stage embryos) decreased with mercury exposure. Trends in size were strongest for the females of the $Gpi\text{-}2^{100/+}$ and $Gpi\text{-}2^{+/+}$ genotypes and those for fecundity were strongest for the $Gpi\text{-}2^{100/100}$ and $Gpi\text{-}2^{100/+}$ genotypes. The clearest differences from reproduction to growth was seen for the $Gpi\text{-}2^{100/+}$ heterozygote.

The trends seen here conform to the notion of a trade-off of growth versus reproduction under stress but an alternate hypothesis confounds interpretation based solely on energy allocation. Size-dependent mortality during mercury exposure could have contributed to the differences seen in standard lengths among genotypes. Actual growth information (growth increments of sagittal otoliths) for the mesocosms suggested little difference with mercury treatment although genotype-specific growth rates could not be measured. The differences in fish length seen in Figure 6.4 could include consequences of size- and genotype-dependent mortality under mercury exposure. This size- and genotype-dependent mortality would be consistent with other work by this group (i.e. Diamond *et al*; 1989, Newman *et al.* 1989; Heagler *et al.* 1993).

Dismissing the size differences from further discussions of energy trade-off context, genotype-dependent decreases in reproductive allocation remain clear with mercury exposure. An inadequate, alternative explanation for differences in fecundity between treatments could be size-dependent fecundity, not an energy trade-off. Fish were generally bigger in the exposed tanks and reproductive allocation in bigger fish may be different from that in smaller fish. However, Mulvey *et al.* (1995) applied analysis of covariance to reject this alternative hypothesis. The genotype-dependent shifts in reproduction were life history responses to mercury exposure. Increased demands on energy resources to individual maintenance during mercury exposure resulted in diminished allocation of resources to reproduction. Genotypes at the *Gpi-2* locus differed in how resource allocation occurred under mercury stress.

This example describes only one component of a larger study of mercury and mosquitofish genetics. Other aspects will be explored in Chapter 8.

Continuous variation in phenotype with environmental change is not the only type of phenotypic plasticity. Polyphenism occurs if an environmental cue triggers expression of one phenotype or another with no intermediate phenotypes being expressed. Two or more distinct phenotypes from one genotype may be produced as a consequence of developmental switching. An *à propos* example of polyphenism is the influence of xenobiotic estrogens on sex determination of slider turtles (Bergeron, Crews and McLachlan 1994). For the red-eared slider (*Trachemys scripta*), polyphenism takes place with nest incubation temperature being the usual cue determining hatchling sex. At a temperature dictating a preponderance of male hatchlings, spotting the shell of developing red-eared slider turtle eggs with a polychlorinated biphenyl (2 ', 4 ', 6 '-trichloro-4-biphenylol) solution dramatically increased the likelihood of a hatchling emerging as a female. The PCB triggered an estrogen-mediated switch responsible for sex determination.

6.2.2 TOXICANTS AND AGING

'The [evolutionary] cost of division into the germ line and soma was death' (Stearns 1992). Binary fission in microbes or clonal reproduction in some metazoans produces essentially immortal lines. For other species such as ourselves, specialization of cell lines to produce somatic and germ cell lines resulted in individuals (soma) with finite life spans. The aging and death of the soma are subject to selection in a rather complex way. Differences in fitness of post-reproductive individuals may be trivial relative to continuance of the germ line; therefore, natural selection will not act strongly on such fitness differences. More than a century ago, Weismann (1882, cited in Medvedev 1990) extended this line of reasoning to suggest that a post-reproductive individual could drain the limited resources available to a population because of competition with individuals still contributing to the germ line. Age-related death removes this impediment to germ line success. Such a situation might result in natural selection against long life after an individual (soma) ceases to contribute to the germ line.

What determines how long an individual can live? People have long been fascinated with how genetic and environmental factors, alone or in combination, dictate longevity. Literally, hundreds of theories and paradigms surround this aspect of life history. Medvedev (1990) argued that no single cause for aging exists and many of the current theories are complementary. Disparate theories will be combined into a more inclusive whole in the near future. For example, the limited life span theory, Gompertz Law, and selection-based theory can easily be combined. The limited life span theory, recently disputed by Curtsinger *et al.* (1992), holds that each individual has a genetically predetermined maximum life span (Brooks, Lithgow and Johnson 1994). Such a powerful, genetic influence on longevity is clear in work by Kenyon *et al.* (1993) who produced a nematode (*Caenorhabditis elegans*) strain that differed by only one gene (*daf*-2) from the wild type but lived twice as long as the wild type. Gompertz Law, also questioned recently (Barinaga 1992; Carey *et al.* 1992), holds that death rate increases inexorably and exponentially with age. Selection-based theory holds that genetic factors favored in young individuals can become disadvantageous as individuals age. An antagonistic pleiotropy exists because there is no selective advantage to sparing older, post-reproductive individuals from harm emerging later from these genetic factors: overall fitness of an individual is determined more by advantageous traits of younger (pre-reproductive or reproductive) individuals than disadvantageous traits of older individuals (Rose and Charlesworth 1980; Parsons 1995). This quick review of the limited life span theory, Gompertz Law, and selection-based theory suggested that all could easily be combined into a complementary whole.

Other theories focus on environmental factors and their influence on longevity. They are directly relevant to understanding phenotypic changes in populations under toxicant stress and contribute to understanding the mechanisms for toxicant effects on aging. The discussion of aging models described below is not inclusive and the reader is directed to Medvedev (1990), Stearns (1992), and Parsons (1995) for more comprehensive reviews.

6.2.2.1 Stress-based Theories of Aging

Parson (1995) extends the limited life span theory to the rate of living theory of aging. A particular genotype has a total metabolic allocation that is fixed: longevity is influenced by how quickly or slowly this metabolic allocation is spent. Supporting this theory is the consistent observation that reduced metabolic rate associated with a calorie-restricted diet increases longevity of rodents (Pieri *et al.* 1992) and some nonmammalian species (Sohal and Weindruch 1996). It follows that toxicant stress can influence longevity because metabolic rate commonly increases with stress. Stress could accelerate expenditure of the organism's fixed amount of energy. Kramer *et al.* (1992) found differences in glycolytic flux in mercury-exposed mosquitofish differing in *Gpi-2* allozyme genotype and correlated them to differential survival during acute exposure. Glycolytic flux increased for the mercury-sensitive genotype but not the other genotypes. In this context, the rate of living theory is generally consistent with the stress theory of aging described next.

Parsons (1995) describes the stress theory of aging. Natural selection occurs for resistance to stress and, as a consequence, individuals most resistant to stress will be those with extreme longevity. Longevity is 'incidental to selection for stress resistance' (Parsons 1995). Evidence supportive of this theory can be found in *Drosophila* populations in which longevity was correlated with low metabolic rate and elevated antioxidant activity.

The correlation of antioxidant activity with longevity noted by Parsons (1995) also supports the oxidative stress hypothesis for aging. Further support is provided by increased free radical production and consequent increased oxidative damage in rodents fed an unrestricted diet in the Pieri *et al.* (1992) study described above. The oxidative stress hypothesis of aging holds that aerobic (and photosynthetic) organisms produce reactive oxygen metabolites (e.g. hydrogen peroxide, H_2O_2, the superoxide radical, $O_2^{\bullet -}$, and the hydroxyl radical, $^{\bullet}OH$) which cause oxidative damage and the accumulation of this oxidative damage is a major factor determining life span. Damage to membranes (via lipid peroxidation), DNA, and proteins causes dysfunction and, in the case of DNA, potential for mutation. 'The basic tenet of the oxidative stress hypothesis is that senescence-related loss of function is due to the progressive and irreversible accrual of molecular oxidative damage' (Sohal and Weindruch 1996). Consequently, chronological age is correlated with cumulative oxidative damage: individuals with different rates of oxidative damage accumulation will possess different longevities.

If the oxidative stress hypothesis is valid, individuals experiencing elevated levels of oxidative stress should age at an accelerated rate. Chemical (e.g. the herbicide, paraquat, polycyclic aromatic hydrocarbons, and several heavy metals) and physical (e.g. asbestos fibers or cigarette smoke) agents enhance production of reactive oxidants, accelerating the accumulation of oxidative damage. Oxyradicals (e.g. alkoxyradicals, $RO^{\bullet}$, and peroxyradicals, $ROO^{\bullet}$ where R indicates some organic compound) produced from xenobiotics during detoxification transformations can cause oxidative damage. Other toxicants, including some metals, are involved in production of reactive oxygen metabolites (i.e. H_2O_2, $O_2^{\bullet -}$, and $^{\bullet}OH$) via the catalyzed Haber–Weiss reaction. Damage can be reduced by production of antioxidants (e.g. glutathione) that react with oxyradicals and by synthesis of enzymes that reduce levels of reactive oxygen metabolites (e.g. glutathione peroxidase, catalase and superoxide dismutase) (Burdon 1999). The suite of responses to oxidative stress, collectively called the oxidative stress response, exhibits phylogenetic variation and is subject to natural selection. Therefore adaptation is possible for moderating the oxidative stress-related aging of exposed individuals.

6.2.2.2 Disposable Soma and Related Theories of Aging

The force of selection decreases with age because an individual's contribution to continuance of the germ line decreases. The soma — the individual — gradually becomes increasingly disposable as it contributes less and less to the germ line. According to the antagonistic pleiotropy hypothesis of aging, pleiotropic genes that have a positive effect on a young individual but a negative effect on an old one are favored by selection, and those with negative effect on young but positive on old are selected against (Hughes and Charlesworth 1994). Consequently, genes positively affecting young and negatively affecting old individuals accumulate through time in species.

According to the mutation accumulation theory of aging, the intrinsic qualities of the soma (e.g. slow accumulation of somatic mutations) combine with the decreasing force of selection as the individual grows older. The accumulation of mutations leads to diminished functioning of individuals, e.g. lowered physiological functioning or enhanced risk of cancer. According to this theory, aging results from (1) specialization of individual's cells into soma or germ line, (2) antagonistic pleiotropy, and (3) accumulation of somatic mutations (Stearns 1992). Toxicants that change the duration of various life cycle stages can influence the timing of these adverse manifestations. This combination of toxicant-modified life cycle timing, antagonistic pleiotropy, and accumulation of mutations can diminish the fitness of exposed individuals.

6.2.3 OPTIMIZING FITNESS: BALANCING SOMATIC GROWTH, LONGEVITY, AND REPRODUCTION

Life history evolution makes the simplifying claim that the phenotype consists of demographic traits — birth, age, and size at maturity, number and size of offspring, growth and reproductive investment, length of life, death — connected by constraining relationships, trade-offs. These traits interact to determine individual fitness. (Stearns 1992)

Given a change in environmental conditions such as the introduction of a toxicant, individuals will reallocate energy resources among essential functions. Perhaps, as suggested by the simple K-rule triage, more resources will be used for maintaining (survival) and less for increasing (growth) the soma. Or, perhaps, a more complex allocation would be set in motion to optimize fitness (e.g. Table 6.2).

Each individual has a certain plasticity in its life history traits that can be invoked but each also has limits to this plasticity that it cannot exceed. Described below are some theoretical schemes for the optimal allocation of energy resources. As an example, an individual undergoing chronic stress that slows growth might decrease its size and age at sexual maturity so that it minimizes any reduction in fitness (Stearns and Crandall 1984) or increase the time between litters (Reznick and Yang 1993). (In this context, the fitness of an individual might be reflected in its reproductive value, i.e. V_A in equation (5.9). Reproductive value incorporates

Table 6.2. Selected Examples of Life History Shifts during Exposure to Diverse Stressors

Stressor	Species	Life history trait shifts	Citation
Plants			
Low moisture, salt, low nutrients	*Spartina patens*	Slow growth rates	Silander and Antonovics (1979)
Heavy metals	*Agrostis capillaris* (Predominantly clonal growth strategy)	Increased vegetative growth of tolerant strains versus sensitive strains grown on contaminated soil	Wilson (1988)
Heavy metals	*Plantago lanceolata*	Slow growth rates	Antonovics and Primack (1982)
Invertebrates			
Thermal	*Asellus aquaticus*	Decreased longevity Bred at younger age and smaller size	Aston and Milner (1980)
Coal mine effluent	*Asellus aquaticus*	Lower investment in reproduction Fewer but larger offspring	Maltby (1991)
Vertebrates			
Heavy metals	*Catostomus commersoni*	Increased growth (length and weight) Increased fecundity (but smaller eggs) Decreased overall reproductive success Decreased age of maturity Decreased longevity	McFarlane and Franzin (1978)
Food limitation	*Poecilia reticulata*	Age of maturity increases Size at maturity and growth rate decrease	Reznick (1990)
		Larger (heavier) offspring Longer period between broods	Reznick and Yang (1993)
High predation on adults	*Poecilia reticulata*	Early maturation	Reznick Brygan and Endler (1990)

Table 6.2. (*Continued*)

Stressor	Species	Life history trait shifts	Citation
		Higher reproductive effort	Reznick Rode and Carenas (1996)
		More but smaller young	
High overall predation	*Poecilia reticulata*	Early maturation at smaller size	Reznick and Bryga (1996)
		More but smaller young	
		Higher reproductive effort	

Table 6.3. Predictions for life history shifts with mortality and growth stress[1]

Stress type	Response
Mortality	1. Increased growth with increasing stress (Sibly and Calow 1989)
	2. Less investment in defense and repair with increasing stress (Sibly and Calow 1989)
	3. Short generation time favored, reducing risk of death between birth and reproduction (Sibly and Calow 1989)
	4. (Adult mortality) Early maturation and increased reproductive effort (Reznick Bryga and Endler 1990)
	5. (Juvenile mortality) Late maturation and decreased reproductive effort (Reznick Bryga and Endler 1990)
Growth	1. Increased growth with increasing stress (Sibly and Calow 1989)
	2. Less investment in defense and repair with increasing stress (Sibly and Calow 1989)

[1] Stress is defined here as anything that reduces the Darwinian fitness of an individual.

both the cumulative production of young and the timing of parturition which affects when young begin contributing to the germ line. The r may be used cautiously to measure the 'fitness' of a lineage or population.) Exactly how individual size and age at maturity change is determined by the constraints on life history plasticity of the species and the genetic constitution of the particular individual.

Several general predictions are made based on life history theory (Table 6.3). An obvious one occurring with increased stress and insufficient phenotypic plasticity would be higher mortality and reproductive failure. As likely as this scenario is, it is a not a life history response: it is a failure to respond. The first two predictions of life history responses are derived directly from Reznick's work with guppies (*Poecilia reticulata*) (Reznick 1990; Reznick, Bryga and Endler 1990) and the third is a more involved scheme emerging from work by Sibly and colleagues (Sibly and Calow 1989; Holloway, Sibley and Povey 1990;

Sibly 1996). First, if environmental conditions tend to increase adult mortality, individuals will shift toward early maturation and increased reproductive effort (Reznick, Bryga and Endler 1990). Second, if environmental conditions increase juvenile mortality, individuals will shift to late maturation and decreased reproductive effort (Reznick, Bryga and Endler 1990). Third and most complex, a juvenile must strike a balance between growth and survival in any stressful environment. If a toxicant presents a high risk of killing the individual outright, the individual will allocate resources to maintain the highest fitness (survival) possible under these conditions. Alternately, the toxicant can impact the individual's production which can be measured as a decrease in its scope of growth. (Scope of growth is the amount of all energy taken in by the individual minus its metabolic losses.) Toxicants can decrease productivity by increasing metabolic losses, e.g. losses due to protein synthesis or turn-over. Sibly and colleagues noted that numerous strategies occur for balancing juvenile growth against survival. A trade-off curve exists and, if in possession of sufficient phenotypic plasticity, individuals will move along that curve to a point of highest fitness for any particular situation.

Sibly and colleagues (Sibly and Calow 1989; Holloway Sibley and Povey 1990; Sibly 1996) visualize life history responses to stress with trade-off curves as shown in Figure 6.5. To use this approach for prediction, an understanding is needed of the species' phenotypic plasticity relative to growth and survival rates, and the general mode of impact for the toxicant on the species. Does the toxicant influence the species by primarily decreasing survival or by decreasing productivity? The trade-off curve will shift upward if mortality stress is present or to the left if growth stress is present (Figure 6.5, middle panel). Sibly and Calow (1989) give the example of a predator as a mortality stressor and lowered ambient temperature for an ectotherm as a simple growth stressor and suggest that many toxicants are likely mixed stressors affecting both, survival and growth. Sometimes, the trade-off curve can change shape with toxicant exposure (Figure 6.5, bottom panel) and confound prediction. If stress doesn't change the shape of the trade-off curve, Sibly suggests that adaptation under mortality or growth stress (middle panel of Figure 6.5) should favor less investment in defense and faster growing individuals (Sibly and Calow 1989). (See Stearns 1992, Table 4.1 for a more detailed matrix of possible life history trade-offs.)

Microevolution is suggested by a change through successive generations toward optimum fitness on the trade-off curves. This process would facilitate a slow shift of phenotypes into a tight cluster around the highest possible fitness value. The result can be microevolution for life history traits, a remarkably fast process in studies of predation (Reznick, Bryga and Endler 1990), habitat stability (Stearns 1983), and toxicant exposure (Maltby 1991).

Several conditions can result in deviations from these predictions. As mentioned, toxicant exposure often changes the shape of the trade-off curve, resulting in predictions other than those highlighted in Table 6.3 for Sibly and

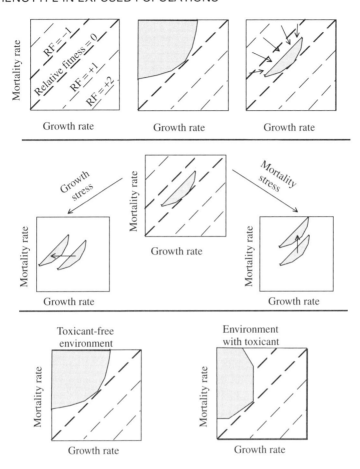

Fig. 6.5. Trade-off curves for life history traits under toxicant stress. The top panel shows lines of identical fitness for various combinations of growth and mortality rates (left box, modified from Figure 1 in Sibly and Calow 1989), the lines of equal fitness plus the range of phenotypes actually possible for individuals in the population (middle box), and the hypothetical shift in phenotypes to optimize fitness (right box) in an unchanging environment. The middle panel shows the shifts in phenotypes (growth and mortality rates) relative to toxicant-induced changes in growth or mortality (Modified from Figures 2 and 10 in Sibly and Calow 1989 and Sibly 1996, respectively). Notice for mortality stress that individuals at the bottom of the shifted crescent have lower mortality, perhaps due to higher investment in detoxification, but slower growth than those at the top of the crescent. The bottom panel shows that the shape of the trade-off curve can change in the presence of the toxicant (Modified from Figure 11 in Sibly 1996)

colleagues (Walker *et al.* 1996). Several tempering points of Stearns (1992) provide a more extensive discussion of possible complicating factors. Energy resources may not be limiting in a particular environment and predictions based on the premise of optimal energy allocation will be invalid. Some trade-offs involve switches, not continuous functions as shown above. Finally, some functions are relatively insensitive to the differences of energy resources in the environment.

Box 6.3   Metals and suckers: effects on life history traits

Life history characteristics of individuals in two white sucker (*Catostomus commersoni*) populations near a base-metal smelter (Flin Flon, Manitoba) were studied relative to their contrasting exposure to metals. Aerial deposition of metals from the Flin Flon smelter to nearby lakes began in 1930 and continued at a high rate until 1974 when installation of a superstack decreased deposition in nearby lakes. Hamell Lake (higher metal loadings) and Thompson Lake (lower metal loadings) were selected based on their contrasting Cd and Zn burdens. Gill nets were set to survey suckers from both lakes, including surveys during the spring spawning. Age was estimated from growth rings of pectoral fin rays with tags being placed on some spawning fish during the first survey to allow verification of this technique. Egg counts were made for subsets of females at the appropriate seasons.

Fish length was similar until age 2 for both lakes. At age 2, Hamell Lake fish began to grow faster than those of the less contaminated Thompson Lake. Adult fish from the more contaminated Hamell Lake were longer than adults from Thompson Lake and generally weighed more than Thompson Lake fish after normalizing weight to fish length. A reduction in life expectancy for the Hamell Lake suckers was suggested as mean ages were 4.3 and 6.2 years for Hamell and Thompson Lake suckers, respectively. Mortality in Hamell Lake occurred earlier in life (prenatal or early larval stage) than in Thompson Lake. Older fish had similar mortality rates (*circa* 0.8/year) in both lakes. Therefore, in general, Hamell Lake suckers grew faster (after year 2), were more rotund, and died earlier than those from Thompson Lake.

Reproductive effort was also distinct for fish from the two lakes. Hamell Lake suckers matured at an earlier age. Mean egg diameter for Hamell Lake fish (1.74 mm) was significantly smaller than for Thompson Lake fish (1.82 mm). Curiously, Hamell Lake females surveyed in June-July of 1976 had not spawned whereas all of Thompson Lake fish had completed spawning. Egg reabsorption for Hamell Lake female suckers was evident. McFarlane and Franzin estimated that Hamell Lake suckers experienced a 50% failure in reproduction in the summer of 1976.

The white sucker population of Hamell Lake might have appeared after a typical survey to be unaffected as it had a fast growth rate, heavy individuals, early sexual maturation, and increased egg production. A closer examination revealed shortened longevity, reduced reproductive success and egg size, and low population density as reflected in catch-per-unit-effort data. Increased juvenile mortality was evident. Only by looking at a suite of individual traits could the extent of effect be evaluated.

6.3 DEVELOPMENTAL STABILITY IN POPULATIONS

Developmental homeostasis refers to the stabilized flow of the developmental trajectory. This stabilized flow has two components: canalization and developmental stability. Canalization is the stability of development in different environments. . . .Developmental stability, in contrast, is the stability of development in the same environment. (Graham *et al.* 1993)

. . .a genotype with a low maintenance requirement can support growth over a wide range of environmental conditions. Furthermore, such individuals should show substantial homeostasis in response to stressful environments and should live longest. Since fluctuating morphological asymmetry, FA, is a measure of homeostasis. . .in various environments. . ., the least asymmetric individuals therefore should live longest. (Parsons 1995)

Population phenogenetics ('the study of genetic and environmental influences on the development of the phenotype' within populations (Zakharov and Graham 1992)) will be explored in this section relative to developmental homeostasis. Developmental homeostasis, or more specifically developmental stability, has been used for decades as a metric of population condition but has only recently been applied in ecotoxicology. Simple, but meaningful, measurements possible for assessing the impact of anthropogenic stressors on populations are described by Zakharov (1990) and Graham *et al.* (1993a–c). A population phenogenetics approach has several advantages for assessment of toxicant effects:

(1) In a discipline preoccupied with complex measurement instrumentation and methodologies (i.e. Medawar's (1982) *idola quantitatis*), a refreshing feature of this approach is that a small ruler and, if the anatomical structures of interest are minute, a dissecting microscope might be the only instrumentation required to take all necessary measurements. Measured anatomical traits may be meristic (i.e. phenotypes are expressed in discrete, integral classes such as number of pectoral fin rays) or continuous (i.e. phenotypes are expressed along a continuum such as length of the fifth pectoral fin ray). However, computer-based, image analysis systems can be applied to questions requiring more sophistication or by ecotoxicologists afflicted by *idola quantitatis*.

(2) Equally remarkable in a field biased toward producing effects data for individuals, information on toxicant effects to populations is acquired with these simple tools.

(3) The approach is so general that it can be used for extremely diverse species, e.g. plants (Graham, Freeman and Emlen 1993a), invertebrates (Graham, Roe and West 1993c), and vertebrates (Ferguson 1986; Leary, Allendorf and Knudsen 1987).

(4) Metrics can potentially be used to detect population degradation before extensive or irreversible damage occurs (Zakharov 1990). As implied by Graham and Parsons above, these studies quantify the diminished capacity to produce a population composed of optimally fit individuals due to some environmental condition such as toxicant exposure.

In contrast to the first part of this chapter where emphasis was optimizing fitness by allocation of energy resources among essential functions, the focus here is fitness consequences of imperfect anatomical development. Of course, assuming that development follows the most energetically favorable path in any given situation (Graham, Freeman and Emlen 1993b), developmental stability could be fit into the above energy allocation framework. Regardless, the focus here is on changes in fitness occurring due to changes in anatomical development, not underlying physiological or biochemical processes.

Developmental stability is the capacity to produce similar anatomical phenotypes ('minimize random accidents of development within a trajectory' (Graham, Freeman and Emlen 1993a)) in a particular environment. Why is developmental stability important? Studies show that deviation outside a certain optimal range of phenotypes results in an individual with lowered fitness. Environmental stressors, including chemical toxicants, can lead to decreased developmental stability.

Developmental stability can be estimated in several ways but fluctuating asymmetry (FA) is the most commonly applied metric for bilaterally symmetrical individuals or structures. Fluctuating asymmetry is simply the random (nondirectional) difference (d) in features measured from the left and right sides of individuals (equation (6.1)) (Figure 6.6). These paired measurements are taken from n individuals in the population. If the distribution of d_i values ($i = 1$ to n) is normal and the mean (equation (6.2)) is zero, the variance of the population (equation (6.3)) is a measure of the level of fluctuating asymmetry in the population:

$$d_i = \text{Measurement}_{\text{right } i} - \text{Measurement}_{\text{left } i} \tag{6.1}$$

$$M_d = \frac{\sum d_i}{n} \tag{6.2}$$

$$\hat{\sigma}^2 = \frac{\sum (d - M_d)^2}{n - 1} \tag{6.3}$$

Differences measured for a sample of individuals are used to estimate deviations from perfect bilateral symmetry in the population. Implied in an increasing

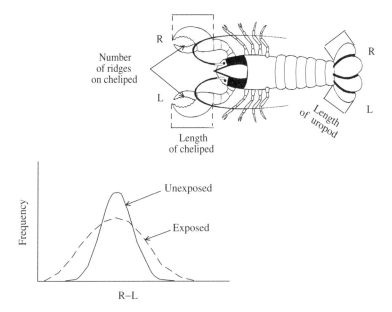

Fig. 6.6. Developmental stability is often measured as fluctuating asymmetry. Morphological features (e.g. length of cheliped or number of ridges on the inside surface of the cheliped) are measured on the right (R) and left (L) sides of individuals with bilateral symmetry. Notice that cheliped or uropod lengths are continuous traits but number of cheliped ridges is a meristic trait. Measurements are made for a sample of individuals from the population and the distribution of differences between R and L measurements used to suggest the level of developmental stability in the population. The larger the variance, the less stable the development. The bottom set of normal curves illustrates the example of more stability in the unexposed population than in the exposed population

FA is a diminished ability to maintain developmental stability — a decline in homeostasis. As a particularly disturbing example, FA for teeth of children born to alcoholic mothers was found to be higher than FA for teeth of children born to nonalcoholic mothers (Kieser 1992). The implication is that *in utero* alcohol exposure caused fetal stress. More relevant to ecotoxicology, Valentine and Soulé (1973) demonstrated increased FA using pectoral fin ray numbers in grunion (*Leuresthes tenuis*) exposed to DDT, suggesting that FA may be a valuable ecotoxicological tool (Valentine, Soulé and Samollow 1973). Several studies have correlated FA with measures of fitness (Parsons 1992; Naugler and Leech 1994; Mitton 1997). Increases in FA were associated with a decrease in Darwinian fitness for individuals in the population. Further, shifts back over several generations from high FA for exposed populations might be evidence for microevolution. Hoffmann and Parsons (1991, p. 107) used laboratory studies showing a drop in FA with stress adaptation of diptera (Mather 1953; Reeve 1960; McKenzie and Clarke 1988) to suggest that such microevolution could occur in the wild.

Fluctuating asymmetry is only one of several asymmetries that can be expressed by bilateral organisms. Directional asymmetry occurs if the mean of the d_i distribution is nonzero. There is a tendency for the asymmetry to be biased to one side. Antisymmetry can occur if there is a bimodal distribution for d_i. The familiar example of antisymmetry is the large claw of adult male fiddler crabs. Males will have a very large claw on the right or left. The result is a bimodal distribution in d_i values for the population. Graham, Freeman and Emlen (1993b) provide a detailed review of these developmental conditions for bilateral organisms or structures.

Box 6.4   Lead, Benzene and Asymmetric Flies

In an unusual ecotoxicological study, Graham, Roe and West (1993c) explored the change in FA of *Drosophila melanogaster* populations exposed to increasing concentrations of lead chloride and benzene. In this laboratory study, these toxicants were added separately to the fly's culture media. Neither lead nor benzene at any concentration affected the number of adult flies produced; however, emergence time was earlier for flies held at the highest benzene concentration (10 000 mg/kg of media) than for flies held at other concentrations.

The numbers of sternopleural bristles on the right and left sides of adults emerging in these treatments were measured. The frequency distribution of differences in the number of bristles was generated for each concentration of each toxicant. The null hypothesis of a mean of zero for d_i values was assessed with t-tests. Conventional tests of normality such as the Shapiro–Wilk's test were not applied. Instead, estimates of kurtosis and skewness were used. An F_{max} test was used to test for significant differences in FA among treatments.

All but one treatment and both toxicants had mean $d(M_d)$ values that were not significantly different from zero. Male fly data for the 10 000 mg/kg benzene treatment were omitted from this analysis because data examination for this treatment indicated directional asymmetry. Although males had fewer bristles than females, the FA for both sexes was similar so FA data were pooled for the sexes. The FA increased significantly ($\alpha = 0.05$) with increasing concentrations of lead or benzene. Figure 6.7 shows the results for both sexes, including the males exposed to 10 000 mg/kg of benzene.

This laboratory study clearly indicates the value of FA as a measure of population consequence of toxicant exposure. Its straightforward design and analysis also shows the ease with which laboratory toxicity tests could be developed for FA, a population-level metric of effect.

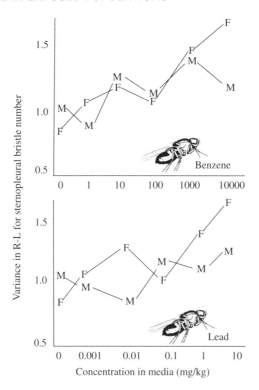

Fig. 6.7. The influence of lead and benzene concentrations in media on the developmental stability of *Drosophila melanogaster* (Data from Table 3 in Graham, Roe and West. 1993b). Sternopleural bristle number was counted on the right and left sides of each individual. M = male and F = female

6.4 SUMMARY

Collusive lying occurs when two parties, knowing full well that what they are saying or doing is false, collude in ignoring the falsity. (Bailey 1991)

Most honest and informed ecotoxicologists would reluctantly admit to participating in a certain level of collusive lying as they assess ecological risk. By applying 96 h LC50, NOEC, MATC, or other values derived from them, risk assessors reluctantly ignore knowledge about populations such as that described here and adhere to the belief that individual-based data are all that are needed to successfully regulate toxicants. This attempt to translate phenotypic variation to population consequences is intended to alleviate some of our dependence on such behavior. Such dependence on clearly false paradigms is as dangerously corrosive to the framework of the science as it is expeditious for environmental regulation.

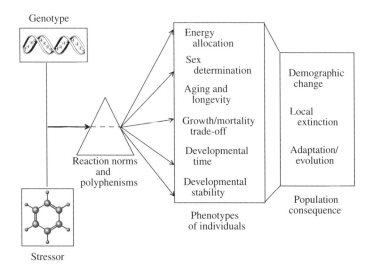

Fig. 6.8. Summarizing the chapter, the genotype of individuals interact with environmental factors, including toxicants, to generate phenotypes. Translation from genotype to phenotype is through reaction norms and polyphenisms. Important life history traits manifested by phenotypes include energy allocation tendencies, sex determination, aging, longevity, trade-offs between growth and survival, rate of development, and developmental stability. The net consequence of changes in life history traits due to toxicant exposure can be demographic change, local extinction, physiological acclimation, and genetic adaptation or microevolution

   The genotype exposed to toxicant can produce a range of phenotypes as described by reaction norms or distinct phenotypes as described by polyphenisms. A spectrum of phenotypes is possible (Figure 6.8) but the range is restricted by inherent limits of each species. Associated changes include those affecting energy allocation, sex determination, aging and longevity, trade-offs between growth and survival, development time, and developmental stability. These traits translate into changes in demographic qualities of populations, likelihood of local population extinction, and potentially, adaptation and microevolution.

6.4.1 SUMMARY OF FOUNDATION CONCEPTS AND PARADIGMS

- The phenotype is a consequence of genetic, environmental, and genetic × environmental factors.
- Changes to individuals can be translated to population consequences by considering processes controlling effects to phenotypes within populations. Theory linkage can occur from physiology → individual life history traits → population phenomena.

- Life history traits of r- and K-strategists under toxicant exposure result in shifts in community composition favoring r-strategists.
- The principle of allocation holds that a finite amount of energy is available to fulfill the diverse life functions of individuals. Rules emerge for the use of energy resources as individuals modify the phenotype to optimize Darwinian fitness.
- Hormesis can be a consequence of energy resource reallocation under low levels of toxicant exposure.
- The reaction norm concept describes phenotypic plasticity relative to life history traits of individuals. Reaction norms transform the variation in an environment to variation in the phenotype.
- Variation in phenotype as a consequence of environmental variation may also involve polyphenism, the production of two or more distinct phenotypes from one genotype.
- Toxicants can influence aging and their influence is consistent with several theories of aging.
- Many theories of aging are not mutually exclusive and will likely be merged into a larger explanatory framework in the future. Some current and toxicant-relevant theories of aging include the limited life span, rate of living, stress-based including oxidative stress, and selection-based theories including the disposable soma theory.
- Trade-offs for life history traits are predicted for individuals under stress as described in Table 6.3 and Stearns's Table 4.1. Trade-offs are complex functions of species characteristics and genetic variation present in the relevant population.
- Developmental stability can be influenced by toxicants. A decrease in developmental stability implies a failure to produce a consistent phenotype in the environment and suggests a reduction in fitness for individuals in the population. Such instability is often measured as fluctuating asymmetry in populations although directional asymmetry and antisymmetry can also be useful.

REFERENCES

Adam SM, Crumby WD, Greeley Jr MS, Ryon MG and Schilling EM (1992). Relationships between physiological and fish population responses in a contaminated stream. *Environ Toxicol Chem* **11**: 1549–1557.

Antonovics J and Primack RB (1982). Experimental ecological genetics in *Plantago*. VI. The demography of seedling transplants of *P. lanceolata. J Ecol* **70**: 55–75.

Aston RJ and Milner GP (1980). A comparison of populations of the isopod *Asellus aquaticus* above and below power stations in organically polluted reaches of the River Trent. *Freshwater Biol* **10**: 1–14.

Atchison GJ, Sandheinrich MB and Bryan MD (1996). Effects of environmental stressors on interspecific interactions of aquatic animals. In *Ecotoxicology. A Hierarchical Treatment*, ed. by MC Newman and CH Jagoe, pp. 319–345. Lewis/CRC Press, Boca Raton, FL.

Bailey FG (1991). *The Prevalence of Deceit.* Cornell University Press, Ithaca, NY.

Barinaga M (1992). Mortality: overturning received wisdom. *Science* **258**: 398–399.

Bergeron JM, Crews D and McLachlan JA (1994). PCBs as environmental estrogens: turtle sex determination as a biomarker of environmental contamination.*Environ Health Perspect* **102**: 780–781.

Bongers T (1990). The maturity index: an ecological measure of environmental disturbance based on nematode species composition. *Oecologia* **83**: 14–19.

Bongers T and Ferris H (1999). Nematode community structure as a bioindicator in environmental monitoring. *TREE* **14**: 224–228.

Brooks A, Lithgow GJ and Johnson TE (1994). Mortality rates in a genetically heterogeneous populations of *Caenorhabditis elegans. Science* **263**: 668–671.

Burdon RH (1999). *Genes in the Environment.* Taylor & Francis Inc., Philadelphia, PA.

Calabrese EJ, McCarthy ME and Kenyon E (1987). The occurrence of chemically induced hormesis. *Health Phys* **52**: 531–541.

Calow P and Sibly RM (1990). A physiological basis of population processes: ecotoxicological implications. *Funct Ecol* **4**: 283–288.

Carey JR, Liedo P, Orozco D and Vaupel JW (1992). Slowing of mortality at older ages in large Medfly cohorts. *Science* **258**: 457–461.

Clark AG (1997). Stress and metabolic regulation in *Drosophila.* In *Environmental Stress, Adaptation and Evolution*, ed. by R Bijlsma and V Loeschcke, pp. 117–132. Birkhäuser Verlag, Basel.

Curtsinger JW, Fukui HH, Townsend DR and Vaupel JW (1992). Demography of genotypes: failure of the limited life-span paradigm in *Drosophila melanogaster. Science* **258**: 461–463.

Deevey ES (1947). Life tables for natural populations. *Q Rev Biol* **22**: 283–314.

Diamond SA, Newman MC, Mulvey M, Dixon PM and Martinson D (1989). Allozyme genotype and time to death of mosquitofish, *Gambusia affinis* (Baird and Girard), during acute exposure to inorganic mercury. *Environ Toxicol Chem* **8**: 613–622.

Ferguson MM (1986). Developmental stability of rainbow trout hybrids: genomic coadaptation or heterozygosity? *Evolution* **40**: 323–330.

Freeman DC, Graham JH and Emlen JM (1993). Developmental stability in plants: symmetries, stress, and epigenetic effects. In *Developmental Stability: Origins and Evolutionary Significance*, ed. by T Markow, pp. 97–119. Kluwer, Dordrecht.

Forbes VE, Møller V, Browne RA and Depledge MH (1999). The influence of reproductive mode and its genetic consequences on the responses of populations to toxicants: a case study. In *Genetics and Ecotoxicology*, ed. by VE Forbes, pp. 187–206. Taylor & Francis, Inc., Philadelphia, PA.

Graham JH, Freeman DC and Emlen JM (1993a). Developmental stability: a sensitive indicator of populations under stress. In *Environmental Toxicology and Risk Assessment, ASTM STP 1179*, ed. by WG Landis, JS Hughes and MA Lewis, pp. 136-158. American Society for Testing and Materials, Philadelphia, PA.

Graham JH, Freeman DC and Emlen JM (1993b). Antisymmetry, directional asymmetry, and dynamic morphogenesis. *Genetica* **89**: 121–137.

Graham JH, Roe KE and West TB (1993c). Effects of lead and benzene on the developmental stability of *Drosophila melanogaster. Ecotoxicology* **2**: 185–195.

Heagler MG, Newman MC, Mulvey M and Dixon PM (1993). Allozyme genotype in mosquitofish, *Gambusia holbrooki*, during mercury exposure: temporal stability, concentration effects and field verification. *Environ Toxicol Chem* **12**: 385–395.

Hickey DA and McNeilly T (1975). Competition between metal tolerant and normal plant populations: a field experiment on normal soil. *Evolution* **29**: 458–464.

Hoffmann AA and Parsons PA (1991). *Evolutionary Genetics and Environmental Stress.* Oxford University Press, Oxford.

Holloway GJ, Sibly RM and Povey SR (1990). Evolution in toxin-stressed environments. *Funct Ecol* **4**: 289–294.
Hughes KA and Charlesworth B (1994). A genetic analysis of senescence in *Drosophila*. *Nature* **367**: 64–66.
Kammenga JE, Van Koert PHG, Riksen JAG, Korthals GW and Bakker J (1996). A toxicity test in artificial soil based on the life-history strategy of the nematode *Plectus acuminatus*. *Environ Toxicol Chem* **15**: 722–727.
Kenyon C, Chang J, Gensch E, Rudner A and Tabtiang R (1993). A *C. elegans* mutant that lives twice as long as wild type. *Nature* **366**: 461–464.
Kieser JA (1992). Fluctuating asymmetry and maternal alcohol consumption. *Ann Hum Biol* **19**: 513–520.
Kooijman SALM (1993). *Dynamic Energy Budgets in Biological Systems*. Cambridge University Press, Cambridge.
Kooijman SALM, Van der Hoeven N and Van der Werf DC (1989). Population consequences of a physiological model for individuals. *Funct Ecol* **3**: 325–336.
Kramer VJ, Newman MC, Mulvey M and Ultsch GR (1992). Glycolysis and Krebs cycle metabolites in mosquitofish, *Gambusia holbrooki*: Girard 1859, exposed to mercuric chloride: allozyme genotype effects. *Environ Toxicol Chem* **11**: 357–364.
Kreuger DA and Dodson SI (1981). Embryological induction and predation ecology in *Daphnia pulex*. *Limnol Oceanogr* **26**: 219–223.
Leary RF, Allendorf FW and Knudsen KL (1987). Differences in inbreeding coefficients do not explain the association between heterozygosity at allozyme loci and developmental stability in rainbow trout. *Evolution* **41**: 1413–1415.
Levins R (1968). *Evolution in Changing Environments*. Princeton University Press, Princeton, NJ.
Locke J (1706). *Of the Conduct of the Understanding*. Reprinted in Grant RH and Tarcov N (eds.) (1996). *Some Thoughts on Education; and, Of the Conduct of Understanding*. Hackett Publ. Co., Inc., Indianapolis, IN.
Maltby L (1991). Pollution as a probe of life-history adaptation in *Asellus aquaticus* (Isopoda). *Oikos* **61**: 11–18.
Mather K (1953). Genetic control of stability in development. *Heredity* **7**: 297–336.
May RM (1976). *Theoretical Ecology. Principles and Applications*. W.B. Saunders Co., Philadelphia, PA.
McFarlane GA and Franzin WG (1978). Elevated heavy metals: a stress on a population of white suckers, *Catostomus commersoni*, in Hamell Lake, Saskatchewan. *J. Fish. Res. Board Can* **35**: 963–970.
McKenzie JA and Clarke GM (1988). Diazinon resistance, fluctuating asymmetry and fitness in the Australian sheep blowfly, *Lucilia cuprina*. *Genetics* **120**: 213–220.
Medawar PB (1982). *Plato's Republic*. Oxford University Press, Oxford.
Medvedev ZA (1990). An attempt at a rational classification of theories of ageing. *Biol Rev* **65**: 375–398.
Mitton JB (1997). *Selection in Natural Populations*. Oxford University Press, Oxford.
Mulvey M, Newman MC, Chazal A, Keklak MM, Heagler MG and Hales Jr LS (1995). Genetic and demographic responses of mosquitofish (*Gambusia holbrooki* Girard 1859) populations stressed by mercury. *Environ Toxicol Chem* **14**: 1411–1418.
Naugler CT and Leech CM (1994). Fluctuating asymmetry and survival ability in the forest tent caterpillar moth *Malacosoma disstria*: implications for pest management. *Entomologia Exp Appl* **70**: 295–298.
Neuhold JM (1987). The relationship of life history attributes to toxicant tolerance in fishes. *Environ Toxicol Chem* **6**: 709–716.
Newman MC (1998). *Fundamentals of Ecotoxicology*. Ann Arbor Press, Chelsea, MI.

Newman MC, Diamond SA, Mulvey M and Dixon PM (1989). Allozyme genotype and time to death of mosquitofish, *Gambusia affinis* (Baird and Girard), during acute toxicant exposure: a comparison of arsenate and inorganic mercury. *Aquat Toxicol* **15**: 141–159.

Odum EP (1985). Trends expected in stressed ecosystems. *Bioscience* **35**: 419–422.

Parsons PA (1992). Fluctuating asymmetry: a biological monitor of environmental and genomic stress. *Heredity* **68**: 361–364.

Parsons PA (1995). Inherited stress resistance and longevity: a stress theory of ageing.*Heredity* **75**: 216 221.

Petersen Jr RC and Petersen LB-M (1988). Compensatory mortality in aquatic populations: its importance for interpretation of toxicant effects. *Ambio* **17**: 381–386.

Pieri C, Falasca M, Recchioni R, Moroni F and Marcheselli F (1992). Diet restriction: a tool to prolong lifespan of experimental animals. Models and current hypotheses of action. *Comp Biochem Physiol* **103**A: 551-554.

Posthuma JF, van Kleunen A and Admiraal W (1995). Alterations in life-history traits of *Chironomus riparius* (Diptera) obtained from metal contaminated rivers. *Arch Environ Contam Toxicol* **29**: 469–475.

Reeve ECR (1960). Some genetic tests on asymmetry of sternopleural chaeta number in *Drosophila*. *Genet Res* **1**: 151–172.

Reznick DN (1990). Plasticity in age and size at maturity in male guppies (*Poecilia reticulata*): an experimental evaluation of alternate models of development. *J Evol Biol* **3**: 185–203.

Reznick DN (1996). Life-history evolution in guppies (*Poecilia reticulata*: Poeciliidae). V. Genetic basis of parallelism in life histories. *Am Nat* **147**: 339–359.

Reznick DN, Bryga H and Endler JA (1990). Experimentally induced life-history evolution in a natural population. *Nature* **346**: 357–359.

Reznick DN, Rodd FH and Carenas M (1996). Life-history evolution in guppies *(Poecilia reticulata*: Poeciliidae). IV. Parallelism in life-history phenotypes. *Am Nat* **147**: 319–338.

Reznick DN and Yang AP (1993). The influence of fluctuating resources on life history: patterns of allocation and plasticity in females guppies. *Ecology* **74**: 2011–2019.

Reznick DN and Bryga HA (1996). Life-history evolution in guppies (Poecilia reticulata: Poeciliidae). V. Genetic basis of parallelism in life histories. *Am Nat* **147**: 339–359.

Rose M and Charlesworth B (1980). A test of evolutionary theories of senescene. *Nature* **287**: 141–142.

Sagan LA (1987). What is hormesis and why haven't we heard about it before? *Health Phys* **52**: 521–525.

Sagan LA (1989). On radiation, paradigms, and hormesis. *Science* **245**: 574–575.

Selye H (1956). *The Stress of Life*. McGraw-Hill, New York.

Selye H (1973). The evolution of the stress concept. *Am Sci* **61**: 692–699.

Sibly RM (1996). Effects of pollutants on individual life histories and population growth rates. In *Ecotoxicology. A Hierarchical Treatment*, ed. by MC Newman and CH Jagoe, pp. 197-223. CRC/Lewis Press, Boca Raton, FL.

Sibly RM and Calow P (1989). A life-history theory of responses to stress. *Biol J Linn Soc* **37**: 101–116.

Silander JA and Antonovics J (1979). The genetic basis of the ecological amplitude of *Spartina patens*. I. Morphometric and physiological traits. *Evolution* **33**: 1114–1127.

Sohal RS and Weindruch R (1996). Oxidative stress, caloric restriction, and aging. *Science* **273**: 59–63.

Stearns SC (1983). A natural experiment in life-history evolution: field data on the introduction of mosquitofish (*Gambusia affinis*) to Hawaii. *Evolution* **37**: 601–617.

Stearns SC (1989). The evolutionary significance of phenotypic plasticity. *BioScience* **39**: 436–445.

Stearns SC (1992). *The Evolution of Life Histories*. Oxford University Press, Oxford.

Stearns SC and Crandall RE (1984). Plasticity of age and size at sexual maturity: a life history response to unavoidable stress. In *Fish Reproduction*, ed. by G Potts and R Wootton, pp. 13–34. Academic Press, London.

Stebbing ARD (1982). Hormesis—the stimulation of growth by low levels of inhibitors.*The Sci Tot Environ* **22**: 213–234.

Svensson E (1997). The speed of life-history evolution. *TREE* **12**: 380–381.

Tatara C, Mulvey M and Newman MC (1999). Genetic and demographic responses of mosquitofish (*Gambusia holbrooki*) populations exposed to mercury for multiple generations. *Environ Toxicol Chem* **18**: 2840–2845.

Valentine DW and Soulé ME (1973). Effect of p,p'-DDT on developmental stability of pectoral fin rays in the grunion, *Leuresthes tenuis*. *Fish Bull* **71**: 921–926.

Valentine DW, Soulé ME and Samollow P (1973). Asymmetry analysis in fishes: a possible statistical indicator of environmental stress. *Fish Bull* **71**: 357–370.

Walker CH, Hopkin SP, Sibly RM and Peakall DB (1996). *Principles of Ecotoxicology*. Taylor & Francis, London.

Watt WB (1986). Power and efficiency as indexes of fitness in metabolic organization. *Am Nat* **127**: 629–653.

Wilson JB (1988). The cost of heavy-metal tolerance: an example. *Evolution* **42**: 408–413.

Woltereck R (1909). Weitere experimentelle untersuchungen über artveränderung, speziell über das wesen quantitativer artunterschiede bei Daphniden. *Verh D Tsch Zool Ges* **1909**: 110–172.

Zakharov VM (1990). Analysis of fluctuating asymmetry as a method of biomonitoring at the population level. In *Bioindications of Chemical and Radioactive Pollution*, ed. by Krivolutsky DA, pp. 187-198. CRC Press/Mir Publishers, Boca Raton, FL.

Zakharov VM (1992). Introduction. *Acta Zool Fennica* **191**: 4–5.

Zakharov VM and Graham JH (1992). Developmental stability in natural populations. *Acta Zoologica Fennica* **191**: 1–5.

7 Population Genetics: Damage and Stochastic Dynamics of the Germ Line

Because they offer neither advantage nor liability, neutral mutations are either lost or fixed by stochastic changes in allele frequency from generation to generation. Thus the evolutionary dynamics of neutral mutations are adequately described by equations employing population size, N, effective population size, N_e, neutral mutation rate, u, and migration rate, m. Neutral theory has had a tremendous impact on population genetics, and many empirical patterns are consistent with predictions arising from neutral theory. (Mitton 1997)

7.1 OVERVIEW

This chapter describes key processes in population genetics other than adaptation and natural selection. To provide a causal context for the remaining chapters, initial discussion outlines how toxicants can damage DNA. The rest of the chapter deals with stochastic dynamics of population genetics. Understanding toxicant effects on stochastic processes is as important as understanding toxicant-driven natural selection.

Qualities of toxicant-exposed populations can be directly influenced by stochastic or neutral processes. 'Neutral' is used here only to indicate genetic processes or phenomena not involving natural selection. Ecotoxicologists often are preoccupied with adaptation via natural selection and, consequently, pay scant attention to neutral processes. At best, neutral processes are invoked as null hypotheses during testing for selection. Current application of such hypothesis tests by ecotoxicologists is notoriously prone to neglect experimentwise Type II errors, i.e. prone to inappropriately favor the 'statistical detection' of selection and reject the neutral theory-based null hypothesis. In the lead chapter of *Genetics and Ecotoxicology* (Forbes 1999), Forbes states 'The ten contributions to this volume address a number of key issues that, taken together, summarize our current understanding of the relationship between genetics and ecotoxicology'. Despite the obvious value of Forbes's book, this statement is as dismaying as it is accurate. Aside from one chapter discussing genotoxic effects, no chapter focuses primarily on neutral processes. Several (e.g. Chapter 4) present discussion of neutral processes but most retain a predominant theme of selection. In contrast, basic textbooks of population genetics (e.g. Crow and Kimura 1970; Ayala 1982;

Hartl and Clark 1989) contain nearly as much discussion of neutral processes as of adaptation and selection.

This preoccupation of ecotoxicologists biases the literature by frequent neglect of obvious alternate explanations for observed changes in exposed populations. To counter this bias and appropriately balance discussion of neutral and selection-based processes, discussion of adaptation and selection will be put off until Chapter 8. Processes leading to a change in the genome, including genotoxicity, will be discussed and then followed by anticipated changes in allele and genotype composition in populations due to genetic drift, population size, isolation, and population structure. Finally, genetic diversity and the potential influence of toxicants are discussed in the context of long-term population viability. Genetic diversity and heterozygosity discussions will create a conceptual bridge to selection-based topics in Chapter 8.

7.2 DIRECT DAMAGE TO THE GERM LINE

Spontaneous and toxicant-induced changes in DNA (mutations) have diverse consequences. Consequences of mutation range from innocuous to minimal to catastrophic relative to individual fitness. Temporal scales of impact on the species population can be immediate (e.g. nonviable offspring from afflicted individuals) or long term (e.g. evolutionary). Effects may be primarily to the soma, as in the case of carcinogenesis, or to the germ line. In this chapter effects to the soma will be neglected and discussions will focus on those to the germ line.

7.2.1 GENOTOXICITY

Genotoxicity, damage to genetic materials by a physical or chemical agent, occurs by several mechanisms but at the heart of most genotoxic events is a chemical alteration of the DNA. This alteration may be associated with free radical formation near the DNA molecule (e.g. radiation damage) or direct reaction of a chemical agent with the DNA. The result is a modified DNA molecule that might not be repaired with absolute fidelity, e.g. base pair changes. DNA damage could result in a single- or double-strand break. Some instances of chromosome damage can even lead to chromosomal aberrations, aneuploidy, or polyploidy. The consequence to the germ line is often an adverse genetic change.

Genotoxicants modify DNA by several mechanisms (Burdon 1999). Some toxicants alkylate the DNA molecule (Figure 7.1). The locations most prone to react with electrophilic alkylating groups are position 2, 3, and 7 nitrogens, and position 6 oxygen of guanine; position 1, 3, 6, and 7 nitrogens of adenine; position 3 and 4 nitrogens and position 2 oxygen of cytosine, and position 3 nitrogen and positions 2 and 4 oxygens of thymine (Burdon 1999).

Monofunctional alkylating agents (e.g. ethyl methane sulfonate in Figure 7.1 or ethylnitrosourea) bind covalently to only one site. Bifunctional alkylating agents

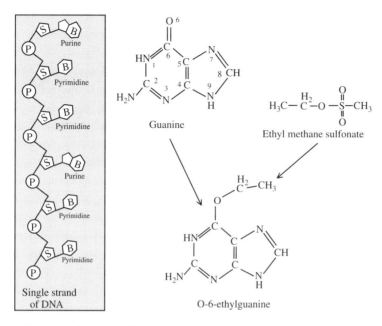

Fig. 7.1. The modification of the purine base, guanine, by the alkylating agent, ethyl methane sulfonate. The DNA molecule (left shaded box: P = phosphate, S = deoxyribose sugar, B = purine or pyrimidine base) is modified at the nitrogenous base by such alkylating agents. Here guanine is covalently linked to an alkylating compound with only one site for potential binding. Guanine alkylated at the position 6 oxygen as shown here often mispairs with thymine and leads to a G:T → A:T transition sequence (Hoffmann 1996). (With a transition, one purine is replaced by another or one pyrimidine is replaced by another.) DNA alkylation can also lead to base loss. For example, an alkyl adduct at position 7 nitrogen of guanine weakens the bond between the base and deoxyribose, and promotes base loss (Hoffmann 1996)

(e.g. sulfur mustards or the antitumor agent, cis-$[PtCl_2(NH_3)_2]$) bind to two sites, potentially crosslinking the two DNA strands. Metabolites of other xenobiotics can also bind to DNA to form adducts, covalently bound additions to the DNA (Figure 7.2). For example, benzo(a)pyrene is rendered more water soluble by a series of phase I detoxification transformations but some products of phase I detoxification (e.g. diol epoxide) readily bind with the nitrogenous bases of the DNA molecule.

Chemicals and ionizing radiation that produce free radicals (Figure 7.3) can modify both the bases and deoxyribose of the DNA molecule. Depending on the nature of the compound or radiation, the result might be a single- or double-strand break in the DNA. As illustrated in Figure 7.3, the reaction with deoxyribose results in a single DNA strand break. Some forms of radiation can release large amounts of energy in short ionization tracks as they pass through tissue and

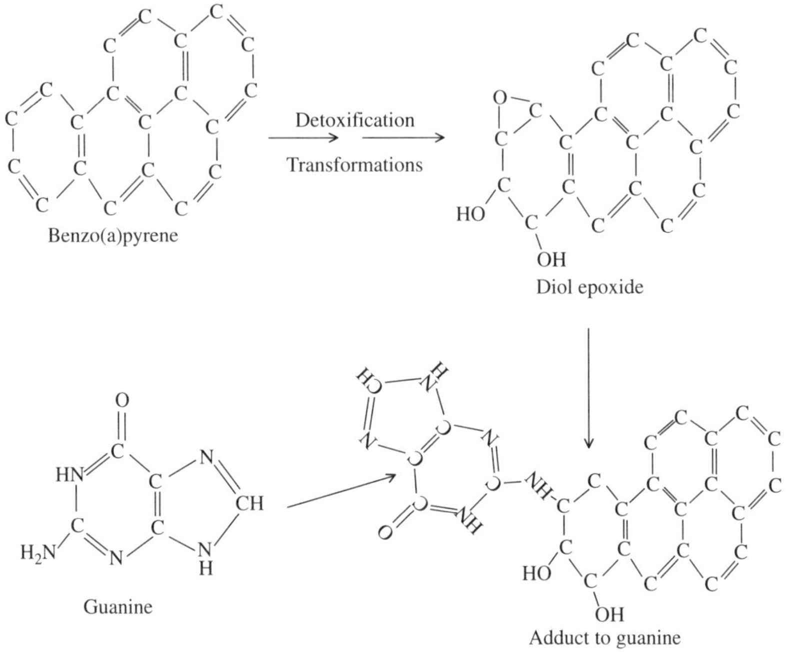

Fig. 7.2. Cytochrome P450 monooxygenase-mediated conversion of the polynuclear aromatic hydrocarbon, benzo(a)pyrene, to a diol epoxide (7b, 8a-diol-9a, 10a-epoxy-7, 8, 9, 10-tetrahydrobenzo (a) pyrene) which forms an adduct by covalently binding to the purine base, guanine. (Modified from Figure 2.5 in Burdon 1999)

interact with water molecules. This results in high local concentrations of free radicals and consequent high levels of breakage in a local region. This increases the chances of a double-strand break. Class b metals such as bismuth, cadmium, gold, lead, mercury, and platinum also bind covalently to N groups in the DNA molecule (Fraústo da Silva and Williams 1993). This binding and associated DNA damage enables the medical use of bismuth, gold, and platinum as antitumor agents. The $Pt(NH_3)_2^{2+}$ of the antitumor agent cis-$[PtCl_2(NH_3)_2]$ avidly binds to DNA by forming two covalent bonds with bases within and between the DNA strands (Fraústo da Silva and Williams 1993). Metals also influence the hydrogen bonding between DNA strands (Figure 7.4) and, because this hydrogen bonding is crucial to proper pairing of complementary bases, can either enhance or reduce the accuracy of base pairings. Metals can also generate free radicals from molecular oxygen via redox cycling and can interfere with transcription of DNA to RNA by binding to associated molecules. All these mechanisms result in varying degrees and types of DNA damage. Although cells have several DNA repair mechanisms, some damage is more readily repaired than others. Mutations

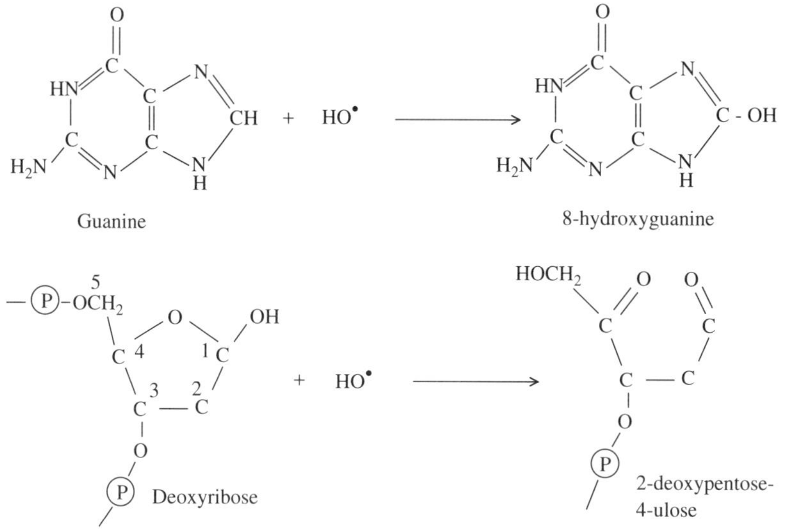

Fig. 7.3. Interaction of the hydroxyl radical with base (guanine) and sugar (deoxyribose) components of the DNA molecule. Notice that the reaction shown with the deoxyribose results in a break in the DNA strand. (Modified from Figures 2.8 and 2.10 in Burdon 1999)

not repaired are perpetuated via the DNA replication process. The result is a wide range of potential modifications to the germ line.

7.2.2 REPAIR OF GENOTOXIC DAMAGE

Several mechanisms for DNA repair and damage-tolerance have been described. For example, pyrimidine dimers formed during exposure to UV light may be enzymatically repaired. Photolyase cleaves these dimers and returns the DNA to its original state. A damage-tolerance mechanism for these dimers allows the replication process to skip over the dimer and proceed normally in its presence. A gap is created in the new DNA strand which is filled in later by repair mechanisms. This process also allows replication and subsequent repair in the presence of damage to occur for DNA adducts.

Alkyltransferases are capable of removing alkyl groups from modified bases, e.g. the ethyl group attached to guanine at position 6 oxygen in Figure 7.1. Burdon (1999) indicates that, because alkyltransferase is inactivated by binding of the alkyl group to cysteine, cells have finite repair capacities. Repair is overwhelmed beyond a certain level of exposure and alkylation damage accumulates. Examples of repair by excision (Bootma and Hoeijmakers 1994) have been described for coping with larger adducts: damaged bases are removed and proper bases are inserted back into the DNA. Also, DNA ligase can insert bases into breaks

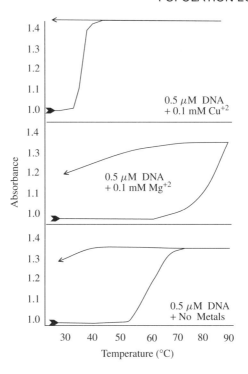

Fig. 7.4. The influence of divalent metals on DNA stability is evidenced by changes in double-/single-stranded DNA composition of DNA solutions that are slowly heated and then cooled. Optical absorbance is low when most of the DNA is present in the double-stranded state and slowly increases as more and more DNA becomes single-stranded. DNA begins to convert to predominantly single-stranded DNA (unwinding) as it is heated without metals to temperatures above *circa* 50°C. It remains as single-stranded DNA as it cools to temperatures below 40°C (bottom panel). The DNA double-stranded structure is stabilized by Mg^{+2}. In the presence of Mg^{+2}, the DNA unwinding occurs at a higher temperature and more DNA reverts to the double-stranded state during cooling. In contrast, the presence of Cu^{+2} results in unwinding at lower temperatures and reversion to double-stranded DNA during cooling is inhibited. The Cu^{+2} clearly interferes with proper base pairing between the strands of the DNA molecule. (Modified from Figure 6.10 in Eichhorn 1974)

in strands. Mismatched bases can be corrected via a mismatch repair process. Hoffman (1996) gives an example of mismatch repair which occurs with deamination of 5-methylcytosine.

These examples should illustrate that diverse types of DNA damage are possible and that a variety of mechanisms for coping with the damage exist. Differences in types of damage and repair fidelities produce differences in genotoxicity among chemicals. For example, DNA damage due to chromium (as chromate) has a lower repair fidelity than that from mercury. Mercury tends to produce single-strand breaks whereas chromate produces more protein-DNA crosslinking. Because single-strand breaks are repaired with higher fidelity than protein-DNA cross-links, chromium is the more carcinogenic of the two metals (Robison, Cantoni and Costa 1984). Similarly, DNA single-strand breaks caused by thallium are repaired less effectively than those from mercury (Zasukhina *et al.* 1983). Imperfect repair can result in mutations within the germ line as well as cancers of the soma. Chronic exposure of male rats to thallium resulted in elevated prevalence of dominant lethal mutations among the embryos they sired (Zasukhina et al. 1983). In contrast, epidemiological studies have found male-mediated genotoxicity associated with Hiroshima atomic bomb survivors to be insignificant (Stone 1992). Indeed, mutation risk is believed to be minor relative to cancer risk in assessing radiation effects to humans (NCRP 1993).

7.2.3 MUTATION RATES AND ACCUMULATION

The natural rate at which mutations appear varies among genes and species. Rates for bacteriophage, bacteria, and vertebrate species range from 4×10^{-10} to 1×10^{-4} mutations per gene per generation (Table 1.4 in Ayala 1982). Mutation rates for humans range from 4.7×10^{-6} to 1×10^{-4} mutations per gene per generation (Table 13-2 in Spiess 1977). Microbes that have no distinct somatic and germ cell lines have mutation rates generally lower than those of metazoans, that is, approximately 10^{-9} to 10^{-6} mutations per cell per replication (Wilson and Bossert 1971).

Hoffmann and Parsons (1997) report that some species respond to increased stress by increasing mutation rates. For example, abrupt upward or downward changes in temperature increase mutation rates of *Drosophila melanogaster*. Jablonka and Lamb (1995) suggest that stress-induced increases in mutation rates may be adaptive because more genetically variable offspring are produced. The likelihood increases for producing an individual better fit to the extreme environment. However, this is viewed as a desperate response to extreme conditions since the likelihood of an adverse mutation increases very quickly too. Here, we will ignore such a response and focus only on increased mutation rate due to DNA damage. Such damage might involve direct genotoxic action or indirect damage, perhaps through increased oxidative stress caused by toxicants or stressors.

Stressors can clearly influence mutation rate in the laboratory and this influence is often dose-dependent (Figure 7.5). However, field demonstrations of stressor-related increases in mutation rates are much less common. Based on sampling of field populations, Baker *et al.* (1996) reported extraordinary base-pair substitution rates for the mitochondrial cytochrome b gene (2.3 to 2.7×10^{-4} versus the anticipated 10^{-6} to 10^{-8} mutations per year) in a species of vole, but later retracted their conclusions based on a lapse in quality control (Baker *et al.* 1997). Convincing evidence from field studies has been reported for increased damage (aneuploidy) in slider turtles (*Trachemys scripta*) exposed to radioactive

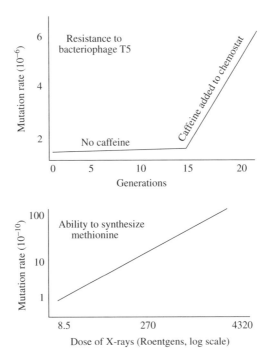

Fig. 7.5. Genotoxic action of caffeine and X-ray irradiation on bacterial mutation rate. Bacteria maintained in a chemostat displayed an abrupt shift in their resistance to bacteriophage T5 after the addition of caffeine to the media (top panel, modified from Figure 7 in Hartl and Clark 1989). Such shifts in mutation rates are often concentration-dependent as evidenced by mutation rates for *E. coli* exposed to increasing doses of X-ray irradiation (bottom panel, modified from Figure 2 in Wilson and Bossert 1971)

contaminants (Lamb *et al.* 1991) and DNA strand breakage for mosquitofish, *Gambusia affinis*, inhabiting radionuclide-contaminated ponds (Theodorakis and Shugart 1999).

7.3 INDIRECT CHANGES TO THE GERM LINE

7.3.1 STOCHASTIC PROCESSES

Stochastic processes can have a strong influence on the genetic composition of a species population. Key stochastic determinants are population size and the spatial distribution of individuals within the population, effective population size, mutation rate, and migration rate. Population size, specifically effective population size (N_e), determines how many individuals are available to carry a particular allele into the next generation. Small populations carry the increased risk of a random loss of an allele if too few individuals are contributing to allele transfer into future generations. Mutation rates, although very low, can influence the long-term genetic diversity of populations. Migration among subpopulations can dramatically influence the risk of allele loss or fixation. These population genetic parameters are explored below in a quantitative manner. However, before doing this, protein and DNA methods applied in the following studies are described briefly in Box 7.1.

Box 7.1   Methods applied in ecotoxicology to define genetic qualities of individuals

Advances in molecular genetic techniques have made the collection of genetic data for toxicological studies relatively easy and cost-effective. A variety of molecular genetic markers (protein and DNA) provide powerful tools to investigate population demographic patterns, genetic variability in natural populations, gene flow, and ecological and evolutionary processes.

Environmental toxicologists are often interested in physiological or biochemical phenotypes, e.g. susceptibility, resistance, or tolerance to toxicants that are not readily assessed at the population level because they may be under the complex control of many genes and may be subject to environmental perturbation. Molecular genetic markers reflect simple genetic underpinnings. Markers may be chosen that behave as neutral markers of population processes or markers thought to be targets for selection can be examined in detail or monitored in populations.

Numerous methods for acquisition of molecular genetic markers are available. Investigators must select from among them the technique that provides the requisite genetic information or variation to address each question (Table 7.1).

Protein electrophoresis

Protein electrophoresis has been used to evaluate population genetic processes in field studies of toxicant impact and in laboratory toxicity studies. Proteins are separated on or in a supporting medium (e.g. starch, polyacrylamide, or cellulose acetate) using an electric field. Specific enzymes or proteins are visualized using histochemical stains. Differences in mobility are associated with charge differences among the proteins. A basic assumption of this method is that these charge differences reflect changes in the DNA sequence encoding the amino acids of the proteins. The bands of activity seen on gels following staining may be isozymes (functionally similar products of gene loci, e.g. GPI-1 and GPI-2) or allozymes (allelic variants of specific loci, e.g. $Gpi\text{-}2^{100}$ and $Gpi\text{-}2^{165}$). Banding patterns are interpreted to be genetically based, heritable, and co-dominant. Interpretation of banding patterns is well established and follows Mendelian inheritance rules.

Table 7.1. A summary of molecular genetic markers and data provided for uses in ecotoxicology

Method	Number of loci	Number of individuals
Protein electrophoresis	Many	Many
RFLP	Few	Many
RAPD	Many	Many
Microsatellites	Few to many	Few to many
DNA sequencing	Few	Few

Protein electrophoresis is a convenient and cost-effective method to obtain information for many loci for many individuals or populations. Detailed descriptions of electrophoretic methods can be found in Richardson, Baverstock and Adams (1986) and Hillis, Mortiz and Mable (1996).

DNA analysis

Nuclear, mitochondrial, or chloroplast genomes may be studied using DNA methods. DNA may be extracted from fresh, frozen, ethanol-preserved, or dried specimens. Gene sequences are routinely obtained by taking advantage of the polymerase chain reaction (PCR). Thermally stable DNA polymerases amplify DNA sequences from small quantities of template DNA. PCR requires short DNA fragment primers to initiate DNA synthesis. Primers can be random or gene-specific.

Restriction fragment length polymorphisms (RFLP) are determined when whole organelle genomes or amplified DNA products are digested with restriction enzymes. Restriction enzymes recognize and cleave double-stranded DNA at specific sites. These sites usually consist of four to six DNA base pairs. Following digestion of DNA with a series of restriction enzymes, the sample is subjected to electrophoresis on agarose gels. The DNA fragments are separated based on their size (number of base pairs). Data consist of the number and size of the resulting fragments. Variation arises from base pair substitutions, insertions, deletions, sequence rearrangements (which may result in the gain or loss of a restriction enzyme cutting site) or differences in overall size of the DNA fragment.

Williams *et al.* (1990) described a method to amplify random, anonymous DNA sequences using PCR. Random amplification of polymorphic DNA (RAPD) uses a single, short primer (approximately 10 bp) for the PCR reaction. PCR products are DNA fragments flanked by sequences complementary to the primer. PCR products are separated by size on agarose or polyacrylamide gels. Data consist of scores of present or absent for the size-separated fragments and, therefore, display a dominant-recessive genetic pattern. Commercially available primer kits make screening for informative markers relatively easy. The RAPD approach is most useful for intraspecific studies.

Microsatellite DNA analysis can provide highly polymorphic multilocus genotype data comparable to that obtained with protein electrophoresis. Microsatellite loci behave as co-dominant Mendelian markers and are useful to evaluate genetic variation within and among conspecific populations. Microsatellite loci are identified by tandem repeats of short (2 to 4 bp) DNA sequences (e.g. CA_n or CTG_n, where n = number of tandem repeats). Changes in the number of repeat units give rise to the scored polymorphism. The PCR technique is used to obtain microsatellites. Microsatellite products are separated by size on agarose or polyacrylamide gels. Difficulties encountered with this technique include the need to screen for polymorphic loci and to develop highly specific primer pairs for the PCR reactions.

Each of the molecular genetic approaches discussed above provides indirect (protein electrophoresis) or incomplete (RFLP) assessment of genetic characteristics. Direct assessment of genetic traits may be obtained with DNA sequencing. The widespread availability of PCR methods and automated DNA sequencers has made this technique increasingly cost-effective. DNA sequencing usually involves larger (20 to 30 bp) specific primers to amplify target sequences. DNA fragments of different lengths are generated using ddNTPs in the PCR reaction for chain termination. Polyacrylamide gels are used to separate the fragments and the base sequence of DNA is determined.

7.3.2 HARDY–WEINBERG EXPECTATIONS

The Hardy–Weinberg principle states that the frequencies of genotypes within populations remain stable through time if (1) the population is a large (effectively infinite) one of a randomly mating, diploid species with overlapping generations, (2) no natural selection is occurring, (3) mutation rates are negligible, and (4) migration rates are negligible. For a locus with two alleles (e.g. alleles designated as 100 and 165) with allele frequencies of p for 100 and q for 165, the genotype frequencies will be p^2 for 100/100, $2pq$ for 165/100, and q^2 for 165/165. For a three-allele locus (e.g. 66, 100, and 165), the genotype frequencies will be r^2 for 66/66, $2rp$ for 66/100, $2rq$ for 66/165, p^2 for 100/100, $2pq$ for 100/165, and q^2 for 165/165. Such a polynomial relationship can be visualized with a De Finetti diagram (De Finetti 1926) (Figure 7.6).

A χ^2 test can be used to test for significant deviation from Hardy–Weinberg expectations,

$$\chi^2 = \sum_{i=1}^{n} \frac{(\text{Observed}_i - \text{Expected}_i)^2}{\text{Expected}_i} \tag{7.1}$$

where n = the number of possible genotypes (e.g. 3 for a two-allele locus or 6 for a three-allele locus), Observed_i = observed number of individuals of the ith genotype, Expected_i = number of individuals of the ith genotype expected

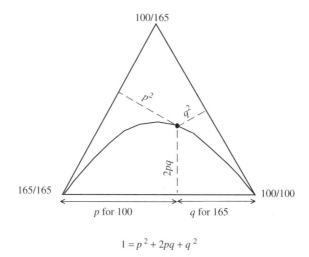

$$1 = p^2 + 2pq + q^2$$

Fig. 7.6. De Finetti diagram illustrating the Hardy–Weinberg principle. Conformity to Hardy–Weinberg expectations for any combination of allele frequencies, e.g. for alleles designated 100 and 165, are indicated by genotype combinations laying on the arc within the 100/100, 165/165, 100/165 triangle. Points off this arc reflect deviations from expectations. The statistical significance of such a deviation can be tested with a χ^2 test

based on the allele frequencies and the Hardy–Weinberg model. The degrees of freedom for the test is the number of possible genotypes minus the number of alleles, e.g. $3 - 2 = 1$ for a two-allele locus.

If the χ^2 test with adequate statistical power failed to reject the null hypothesis, the conclusion is made that there is no evidence that the conditions for Hardy–Weinberg equilibrium were not met. If the null hypothesis were rejected, one or more of the assumptions was violated. As a word of warning, too often ecotoxicologists assume that rejection of the null hypothesis indicates that selection is occurring and ignore the other assumptions upon which the Hardy–Weinberg relationship is based. Such studies must be read with caution.

7.3.3 GENETIC DRIFT

Genotype frequencies do change in populations because of finite population size, population structure, migration, and nonrandom mating. An often-observed consequence of toxicant exposure is a decrease in population size. Population migration rates or direction of migration can be influenced by toxicant avoidance increasing emigration or increased immigration after the toxicant removes a portion of the endemic population and presents vacant habitat to migrating individuals. Population structure can be influenced as toxicants create barriers, impediments, or disincentives to movement, e.g. patches of highly contaminated sediment or a large contaminant plume in a river or stream.

7.3.3.1 Effective Population Size

Genetic drift occurs in all finite populations. Drift can be continuous if the population is always small or intermittent if the population size fluctuates widely. Intermittent drift can produce genetic bottlenecks during times of small population sizes. Due to sampling error, a small population producing future generations will likely carry only a subset of the total genetic variability present in the parent population.

Genetic drift will accelerate as the number of individuals contributing genes to the next generation (effective population size, N_e) decreases. This fact can be illustrated with a simple, random sampling experiment. Assume that a bowl is filled with 5000 red and 5000 blue marbles. We take 5000 marbles randomly from the bowl to produce the 'next generation'. We do this random sampling experiment 1000 times and get an average red:blue ratio each time. With these large numbers, a frequency of red marbles of 0.50 is expected with a modest amount of variation among the 1000 trials. Our sample size is so large that sampling error will be minimal. However, if we sampled only 10 marbles each time, the variation around 0.50 would be much wider than when we sampled 5000 marbles. In fact, in many more cases, the frequency will shift drastically to produce a 'next generation' with a very different frequency of red or blue marbles than that of the 'parent' generation. Indeed, there would be many more cases in which only red or only blue marbles were available to produce the next generation. Drift in frequency of marble color through generations could be simulated by using the new 'generational' frequency from 10 marbles to fill the bowl again with 10 000 red and blue marbles, and repeating the experiment for many generations. Clearly, the sampling error associated with taking only 10 marbles each 'generation' would result in a drift in frequency away from that for the original bowl of marbles. In some cases, blue marbles might be lost completely with fixation occurring for 'red'. The opposite with fixation for 'blue' would occur in other cases. Further, as the frequency of one allele (e.g. frequency of red marbles in the bowl) decreases, the risk of that allele (color) being lost from the population also increases. With intermittent drift and associated bottlenecks, populations can experience founder effects (a population started by a small number of individuals will differ genetically from the parent population due to high sampling error). Small populations bring to future generations a random subset the alleles present in a parent population and allele frequencies vary stochastically from those of the parent population.

The effective population size (N_e) is often smaller than the actual or census population size because all individuals do not contribute to the next generation. How many contribute to the next generation is a complex function of demographic and life history qualities. In general, N_e for a population with nonoverlapping generations is estimated as the harmonic mean of population sizes measured at a series of times (N_i) and the number of generations over which the population measurements were made (t) (Hartl and Clark 1989):

$$\frac{1}{N_e} = \left[\frac{1}{t}\right]\left[\frac{1}{N_1} + \frac{1}{N_2} + \cdots + \frac{1}{N_t}\right] \tag{7.2}$$

The advantage of this estimate of N_e is that it weighs generations with small population sizes more heavily than those with larger populations sizes. Genetic drifts accelerates in a nonlinear manner as population size decreases so this heavy weighting of smaller population sizes is appropriate.

Effective population size is also influenced by sex ratio. As is evident from the use of the harmonic mean again in equation (7.3), the sex present in the lowest number has the most influence on the estimated N_e. If the number of females and males were not equal in the population, the effective population size can be estimated with equation (7.3) or equation (7.4) which is a rearrangement of equation (7.3) (Crow and Kimura 1970):

$$\frac{1}{N_e} = \frac{1}{4N_{\text{Males}}} + \frac{1}{4N_{\text{Females}}} \tag{7.3}$$

$$N_e = \frac{4N_{\text{Males}} \, N_{\text{Females}}}{N_{\text{Males}} + N_{\text{Females}}} \tag{7.4}$$

The 1/4 values in equation (7.3) come from the fact that 'the probability that two genes in different individuals in generation t are both from a male [or female] in generation t-1 is 1/4; and that they come from the same male [or female] is $1/4N_{\text{male}}$ [or $1/4N_{\text{female}}$]' (Crow and Kimura 1970).

If generations are overlapping in time, the assumption $N_e \approx N/2$ can be made or equation (7.5) can be applied:

$$N_e = \frac{4N_a L}{\sigma_n^2 + 2} \tag{7.5}$$

where N_a = the natality over a period of time, L = the mean generation time, and σ_n^2 = the brood size variance.

Genetic drift would eventually lead to loss or fixation of an allele in the absence of an effectively infinite population. How quickly or slowly this occurs is a function of N_e and the initial frequency of the allele in question. Equations (7.6) and (7.7) estimate the average number of generations needed to reach allele fixation ($p \rightarrow 1$) or loss ($p \rightarrow 0$), respectively. Wilson and Bossert (1971) grossly estimate that alleles are lost at a rate of 0.1 to 0.01 per locus per generation if N_e is 10 to 100, 0.0001 per locus per generation if N_e is approximately 10 000, and that loss is insignificant if N_e is greater than 100 000. Ayala (1982) suggests that random drift is unlikely to determine allele frequencies if $4Nx$ is very much smaller than 1 (x = rate of mutation (u), rate of migration (m), or the selection coefficient (s)). (The m is estimated as the number of individuals migrating/total number of individuals that potentially could migrate; the rate of mutation is defined as the number of mutations expected per gamete per generation; the selection coefficient will be defined in Chapter 8.) Values of $4Nx$ greater than 1 implies that mutation, migration and/or selection will dominate changes in allele frequencies. Regardless, excluding times in which the allele is lost, the average number of generations to fixation ($p \rightarrow 1$) for an allele is the following:

$$\bar{t}_1 = -\frac{1}{p}[4N_e(1-p)\ln(1-p)] \tag{7.6}$$

Alternatively, excluding the times when the allele becomes fixed, the average number of generations to allele loss ($p \rightarrow 0$) is the following:

$$\bar{t}_0 = -4N_e \left[\frac{p}{1-p}\right] \ln p \tag{7.7}$$

Crow and Kimura (1970) extend these equations to consider the case of a (neutral) mutation that appears in an individual within a population. (The allele frequency, p, is set to $1/(2N)$ to derive these relationships.) Equations (7.6) and (7.7) become equations (7.8) and (7.9), respectively. The probability of a neutral allele becoming established in the population increases as N_e decreases. Excluding cases in which it is lost from the population, a neutral mutant takes about $4N_e$ generations to reach fixation:

$$\bar{t}_1 \approx 4N_e \tag{7.8}$$

$$\bar{t}_0 \approx 2 \left[\frac{N_e}{N}\right] \ln(2N) \tag{7.9}$$

Why are the above details important to population ecotoxicology? First, the genetic composition of a population can be strongly impacted by a toxicant's influence on the effective population size. The toxicant can influence N_e by decreasing the total population size (equation (7.2)) through time, affecting the numbers of each sex present at any time (equations (7.3) and (7.4)), or modifying generation time or variance in brood size (equation (7.5)). Accelerated drift, genetic bottlenecks, and founder effects can result in loss of genetic information and produce strong shifts in genetic composition of populations (equations (7.6) and (7.7)). If a mutation appears in an individual in a population, its chance of fixation increases as N_e decreases. It might be helpful to reemphasize at this point in our discussions that natural selection has nothing to do with these potential changes in the germ line. Nevertheless, toxicant exposure can led to microevolution because allele frequencies have changed.

7.3.3.2 Genetic Bottlenecks

Drastically reduced population or subpopulation size due to toxicant exposure can result in a genetic bottleneck and consequent founders effect (Newman

1995, 1998; Gillespie and Guttman 1999). An acute toxic exposure, such as that associated with pesticide spraying and subsequent very high mortality, is the most straightforward example of an ecotoxicological event that could result in a bottleneck. Low levels of genetic variation among cheetah (O'Brien *et al.* 1987), Florida panther (Facemire, Gross and Guillette 1995), Lake Erie yellow perch (Strittholt, Guttmann and Wissing 1988), and Great Lakes brown bullhead (Murdoch and Hebert 1994) have been attributed to genetic bottlenecks. The last three examples putatively involved toxicant exposures. The underlying concern associated with bottlenecks is the potential loss of genetic information. Genetic variation in the short term may be associated with physiological or biochemical flexibility and, in the long term, with evolutionary potential and persistence in a changing environment. As an example, conservation biologists are concerned about the ability of the remaining wild cheetahs to cope with a serious infectious disease, feline distemper.

There is a lower, but finite, chance that a population experiencing a bottleneck will emerge with more genetic variation than the parent population because the variation among bottlenecked populations increases as N_e decreases. Whether the genetic variation increases or decreases simply depends on which individuals happen to make it through the bottleneck. However, the chances of a decrease are greater than those of an increase, especially with repeated or periodic bottlenecks, as might be associated with occasional or accidental release of toxicants. Gillespie and Guttman (1999) discussed this possibility of an increase in genetic variation following toxicant exposure but cautioned that maladaptive combinations of rare alleles have a higher chance of occurring in such cases.

7.3.3.3 Balancing Drift and Mutation

From our discussions to this point, the question might arise why genetic drift does not result in a gradual trend toward genetic uniformity. That would be the eventual fate of populations in the absence of mutation. Let's examine the balance between drift and mutation rates by assuming that the relevant genes are neutral. In Chapter 8, we will add details associated with differences in fitness among genotypes.

As mentioned above, the rate of change in a population of N diploid individuals due to a mutation is $2Nu$ and that associated with drift is defined by equations (7.6) to (7.9) and the associated text. The number of novel mutant alleles (M) that appear during each generation, eventually to become fixed, is defined by Spiess (1977):

$$M = \frac{2N\bar{u}}{2N} = \bar{u} \tag{7.10}$$

where $\bar{u}$ = the average of the mutation rates for all alleles. Mutation rate (u) balanced against loss due to genetic drift $(1/(2N))$ results in a steady-state level of genetic variation. Again, this explanation for the maintenance of genetic variation is conditional on neutrality of alleles. Crow and Kimura (1970) and Mitton (1997) indicate that effective population size (N_e) and mutation rate (u) determine the average heterozygosity of a population at equilibrium between the influences of genetic drift and mutation rate: $\overline{H} \approx (4N_e u)/(4N_e u + 1)$. Here, $\overline{H}$ is the average of the $2pq$ proportions for all scored loci where p and q are the allele frequencies for two allele loci. Obviously, the calculation is modified to include loci with more than two alleles. Populations should be expected to differ in their levels of heterozygosity. Some differences could reflect the influence of toxicant exposure on N_e, and perhaps, u.

7.3.4 POPULATION STRUCTURE

What are the genetic consequences of population structure? Generally, an uneven distribution of individuals suggests nonrandom mating; therefore, N_e will be influenced by population structure. Hartl and Clark (1989) indicate that the density of breeding individuals in an area (δ) and the amount of dispersion between an individual's location of birth and that of the birth of its progeny (σ^2) influence N_e:

$$N_e = 4\pi\delta\sigma^2 \qquad (7.11)$$

Clearly, a quality as basic as N_e is strongly influenced by population structure. Other important qualities are discussed in detail below as they often are neglected in ecotoxicological studies.

7.3.4.1 The Wahlund Effect

The Wahlund effect occurs after mixing of populations, each with distinct allele frequencies and in Hardy–Weinberg equilibrium. Mixing may occur during sampling if population structure were cryptic, i.e. individuals were unintentionally taken from two subpopulations and then pooled for analysis. Mixing may occur naturally if migration were taking place between subpopulations previously isolated by a barrier to movement. The frequency of the heterozygote in the mixed sample will be lower than predicted under the assumption that the sample came from a single, randomly mating population. For example, assume that equal numbers of individuals are mixed together from two populations with allele (100, 165) frequencies of $p_1 = 0.9$, $q_1 = 0.1$ and $p_2 = 0.1$, $q_2 = 0.9$. In Hardy–Weinberg equilibrium, the frequencies of the 100/100, 100/165, and 165/165 genotypes in these two populations would be the following:

Population 1 : $p_1^2 = 0.81$ $2p_1q_1 = 0.18$ $q_1^2 = 0.01$

Population 2 : $p_2^2 = 0.01$ $2p_2q_2 = 0.18$ $q_2^2 = 0.81$

Let's assume that 100 individuals from each population were mixed into a pooled sample. From population 1, there would be 81 100/100 individuals,

18 100/165 individuals, and 1 165/165 individual. From population 2, there would be 1 100/100 individual, 18 100/165 individuals, and 81 165/165 individuals. Therefore, the number of individuals of each genotype in the pooled sample would be the following: 100/100 = 82 individuals, 100/165 = 36 individuals, 165/165 = 82 individuals. In the pooled sample, $p(\overline{p})$ and $q(\overline{q})$ values are 0.5 each. The expected number of each genotype predicted from the Hardy–Weinberg principle $(1 = p^2 + 2pq + q^2)$ would be the following: 100/100 = 50 individuals, 100/165 = 100 individuals, and 165/165 = 50 individuals. There is an apparent excess of both homozygotes or, stated another way, an apparent deficit of heterozygous genotypes. Figure 7.7 is a modified De Finetti diagram that visually illustrates this principle.

These same consequences arise if more than two populations are involved. Under conditions giving rise to the Wahlund effect (mixing of individuals from several populations and sampling before reproduction), the average frequency of heterozygotes can be generally described based on the $\overline{p}$ and $\overline{q}$ for a mixed sample involving k populations (Cavalli-Sforza and Bodmer 1971). (Assume equal numbers of individuals being contributed by each of the k populations to the sample.)

$$\overline{H} = 2\overline{p}\,\overline{q}\left[1 - \frac{\sigma^2}{\overline{p}\,\overline{q}}\right] \qquad (7.12)$$

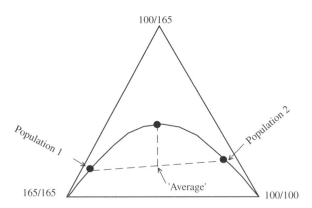

Fig. 7.7. De Finetti diagram illustrating the Wahlund principle. In this example, equal numbers of individuals from two populations are mixed, resulting in an 'average' for the genotype frequencies, 100/100, 100/165, and 165/165. The position defined by these genotype frequencies is off the arc representing all possible solutions to the Hardy–Weinberg polynomial, $1 = p^2 + 2pq + q^2$. The point on the arc immediately above the average reflects the expected frequencies of the three genotypes. Based on these expectations, there is an apparent deficiency of heterozygotes. (Modified from Hartl and Clark 1989)

where σ^2 is the variance in gene frequencies among k populations:

$$\sigma^2 = \frac{\sum p_i^2}{k} - \overline{p}^2 \qquad (7.13)$$

The deficiency of heterozygotes will be roughly twice the σ^2 (Cavalli-Sforza and Bodmer 1971).

Selander's D (Selander 1970) is a straightforward measure of the deviation from expectations. Selander's D is equal to the $H_{obs} - H_{exp}$ where H_{obs} is the observed proportion of heterozygotes in the sample and H_{exp} is the expected proportion of heterozygotes in the sample based on Hardy–Weinberg expectations. A negative D indicates a deficit of heterozygotes.

Samples produced by pooling individuals from several groups of a cryptically structured population might lead the unwary ecotoxicologist to conclude that the heterozygote was less fit than the two homozygotes and underrepresented in the sampled population due to selection associated with toxicant exposure. Such a conclusion must be considered conditional until the possibility of a Wahlund effect was explored carefully.

Box 7.2   Midges, mercury, and too many missing heterozygotes: evidence of a Wahlund effect

Woodward, Mulvey and Newman (1996) examined allozyme frequencies in midge, *Chironomus plumosus*, larvae from Clear Lake (California). Midges of this species emerge as adults to form mating swarms over the lake. Masses containing hundreds of eggs each are deposited on the lake surface by females and the hatched larvae drop to the bottom to become deposit feeders.

Samples of larvae were taken along a transect beginning at the Sulphur Bank Mercury Mine where mine tailings had been deposited in the lake for many decades. Six sites on the transect were sampled by boat using an Eckman dredge. Dredge samples were taken at each site until ample numbers of larvae were collected. Forty midges were deemed an adequate sample for an allozyme survey. On average, chironomids from approximately ten dredge hauls were pooled to obtain the sample size of 40 midges per site.

Twelve polymorphic loci were examined by starch gel electrophoresis (see Figure 7.8 for an illustration) at the six sites; therefore, 72 χ^2 tests for deviation from Hardy–Weinberg expectations were performed. Based on an α of 0.05, only three or four 'false' rejections of the null hypothesis (i.e. Type I errors) would have been expected to occur by chance alone. A surprisingly high proportion of the tests (18 of 72) resulted in the rejection of the null hypothesis. One or more assumptions of Hardy–Weinberg equilibrium was being violated. In 16 cases, Selander's D values were negative, indicating that rejection was associated with a lower than expected proportion of heterozygotes. A review of the sampling methods and egg depositing behavior of the midge suggested a Wahlund effect. Approximately ten dredge samples were taken as the anchored boat drifted over the site. Perhaps individuals pooled from these dredge samples reflected cryptic population structure at each site. Small-scale population structure could result from nonuniform settling of larvae from egg masses, aggregation of siblings, differences in settling behavior relative to sediment characteristics, or some other factor. The alternate explanation of selection at several loci was judged to be less likely than a Wahland effect based on Ockham's razor (i.e. all else being equal, the explanation requiring the fewest assumptions is the most likely) because it requires that selection is occurring against heterozygotes at nine of 12 loci. Explanation based on the Wahlund effect requires only one assumption: the population is structured. In further support of this conclusion, deviations from Hardy–Weinberg expectations that might suggest the presence of selection were not correlated with the level of mercury contamination in site sediments.

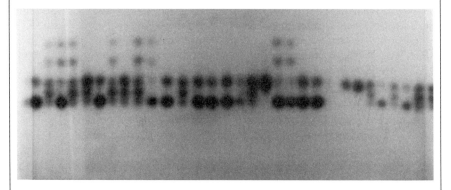

Fig. 7.8. A starch gel stained to score allozymes, allelic variants of enzymes. Supernatants from tissue homogenates are loaded into slots in the gel. Many lanes can be loaded in each gel so that several individuals can be scored on a single gel. After protein separation in an electric field, gels are stained for specific enzyme activities and presumptive genotypes scored based on the pattern of spots in each lane. This particular gel is stained for the enzyme, isocitrate dehydrogenase (*Icd-2* and *Icd-2*), from the tissue of 30 mosquitofish (*Gambusia holbrooki*)

Woodward *et al.*'s study will be explored further (Box 7.3.) after discussion of ways to quantify structuring of populations.

7.3.4.2 Isolated and Semi-isolated Subpopulations

Violations of the assumption for the Hardy-Weinberg model due to nonrandom mating can lead to a deficit of heterozygotes, e.g. the Wahlund effect which appears during sampling of structured populations. Inbreeding can also result in deficits of heterozygotes: an individual's heterozygosity measured as the proportion of all scored loci for which the individual is heterozygous will be lower than its parents if those parents were sibs. The less extreme structuring described to this point is similar to inbreeding because individuals within the total population are not randomly mating due to the degree of their isolation by geographic distance. Population structuring will lead to a decrease in heterozygosity for individuals within a subpopulation relative to that anticipated in the absence of population structure.

The proportion of all individuals that are heterozygotes for a particular locus can be quantified at different levels of 'pooling' to get an understanding of the nature of population structure. The assumption is made that, like increased inbreeding, increased structure in populations results in a decrease in the proportion of individuals that are heterozygotes. Wright's F-statistics (Wright 1943, 1951; Nei 1973) are based on consideration of heterozygosity at the individual (I), subpopulation (S), and the total population (T) levels. Individuals are sampled from subpopulations of the total population to generate the associated metrics, e.g. fish are sampled from creeks and tributaries of a large river system. The heterozygosity estimated at the individual level (H_I) is the observed heterozygosity averaged over all sites, i.e. all subpopulations of the population. The heterozygosity for the subpopulations (H_S) is estimated under the assumption that individuals in the subpopulations are mating randomly, i.e. using $2pq$ estimated for each subpopulation. The total heterozygosity (H_T) is that measured after pooling all individuals from all samples, calculating total p and q values, and estimating the predicted proportion of heterozygotes, i.e. $2pq$ for the entire population. Hartl and Clark (1989) give the following formulae to calculate H_I, H_S, and H_T:

$$H_I = \sum_{i=1}^{k} \frac{H_i}{k} \tag{7.14}$$

where H_i = the heterozygosity for subpopulation i, and k = the number of subpopulations (e.g. sites or sampling locations) from which heterozygosity was estimated.

$$H_S = 1 - \sum_{i=1}^{k} p_{i,s}^2 \tag{7.15}$$

where $p_{i,s}$ = the frequency of allele i for the subsample or site, s:

$$H_T = 1 - \sum_{i=1}^{k} \overline{p}_i^2 \tag{7.16}$$

where $\overline{p}_i$ = allele i's frequency averaged over all subsamples or sites.

Three hierarchical F statistics can be generated from H_I, H_S, and H_T to suggest the influence of population structure on the genotype frequencies at a locus. The F-statistics scale the estimated heterozygosity at the levels of individual, subpopulation, and population. Recalling our discussion linking inbreeding effects and population-structuring effects on heterozygosity, it becomes obvious that several of these metrics are comparable to inbreeding coefficients. The overall inbreeding coefficient, F_{IT}, is defined by equation (7.17) using H_T and H_I from equations (7.16) and (7.14). It is the 'reduction in heterozygosity of an individual relative to the total population' (Hartl and Clark 1989). It quantifies heterozygosity of the individual (H_I) relative to that of the entire population (H_T):

$$F_{IT} = 1 - \frac{H_I}{H_T} = \frac{H_T - H_I}{H_T} \tag{7.17}$$

Similarly, the reduction in heterozygosity of an individual due to nonrandom mating within its subpopulation (equation (7.18)) or due to genetic drift (equation (7.18)) can be derived. The F_{IS} statistic quantifies the heterozygosity of the individual (H_I) relative to that of the (average) subpopulation ($\overline{H}_S$) whereas F_{ST} quantifies the heterozygosity of the (average) subpopulation ($\overline{H}_S$) relative to that of the total population (H_T):

$$F_{IS} = 1 - \frac{H_I}{\overline{H}_S} = \frac{\overline{H}_S - H_I}{\overline{H}_S} \tag{7.18}$$

$$F_{ST} = 1 - \frac{\overline{H}_S}{H_T} = \frac{H_T - \overline{H}_S}{H_T} \tag{7.19}$$

where $\overline{H}_S$ = the average of the H_S values from all subpopulations or sites. The $F_{ST} = 0$ if all subpopulations (e.g. sites) were in Hardy–Weinberg equilibrium. In cases where migration among subpopulations produces deviations from these expectations, F_{ST} is approximately equal to $1/(1 + 4Nm)$ (Rousset and Raymond 1997). Therefore, the effective number of migrants per generation (Nm) can be estimated if F_{ST} is known (Bossart and Prowell 1998). (Note that Ouborg, Piquot and van Groenendael (1999) described Markov Chain Monte Carlo (Beerli 1998), Bayesian (Rannala and Mountain 1997), maximum likelihood (Beerli and Felsenstein 1999), and pseudomaximum likelihood (Rannala and Hartigan 1996) methods that are more effective than this F_{ST}-based methods for estimating effective migration and, in some cases, population structure from molecular genetics data.)

Box 7.3 More on midges, mercury, and missing heterozygotes

In Box 7.2 the potential for a Wahlund effect was identified for a survey of midge allozymes sampled along a gradient of sediment mercury contamination (Woodward, Mulvey and Newman 1996). Differences were tentatively assigned to a Wahlund effect for reasons described in Box 7.2. Wright's F_{IS}, F_{IT}, and F_{ST} statistics were calculated for twelve loci sampled along the mercury gradient in order to understand the observed differences in heterozygosity. A summary for Wright's F-statistics for the following twelve isozymes is provided in Table 7.2: aspartate aminotransferase (*Aat*), adenosine deaminase (*Ada*), esterase (*Est*), glyclleucine peptidase (*gl*), hexokinase (*Hk*), isocitrate dehydrogenase (*Icd-1* and *Icd-2*), leucylglycylglycine peptidase (*lgg*), malate dehydrogenase (*Mdh*), malic enzyme (*Me*), mannose-6-phosphate isomerase (*Mpi*), and phosphoglucomutase (*Pgm*). A quick glance at this table shows that the deficiencies in heterozygotes for many loci were associated with the site (subpopulation, F_{IS}) level. This supports the explanation that sampling of cryptically structured populations produced the apparent deficiency in heterozygotes, i.e. a Wahlund effect. Selection remained an unlikely explanation for reasons discussed in Box 7.2. Inbreeding was another potential mechanism but the lack of any obvious barriers to adult mating as they swarm above the water surface does not support this explanation.

Table 7.2. F_{IS}, F_{IT} and F_{ST} statistics for chironomid larvae collected at six sites along a sediment-associated mercury gradient in Clear Lake (California). Modified from Table 2 of Woodward, Mulvey and Newman (1996)

Allozyme	F-statistic		
locus	F_{IS}	F_{IT}	F_{ST}
Aat	0.165	0.181	0.019
Ada	0.107	0.114	0.007
Est	0.231	0.248	0.022
gl	0.078	0.087	0.010
Hk	−0.116	−0.099	0.015
Icd-1	0.219	0.225	0.009
Icd-2	0.259	0.275	0.022
lgg	0.128	0.130	0.003
Mdh	−0.059	−0.026	0.031
Me	0.618	0.627	0.023
Mpi	0.142	0.151	0.011
Pgm	0.107	0.116	0.010
Mean	0.125	0.137	0.014

To assess this population structure-based hypothesis further, fine-scaled sampling was done at one lake site. Forty larvae were sampled from each of fifteen adjoining, 1 × 1 meter quadrats and scored for nine isozymes (*Aat, Ada, Est, gl, Hk, Icd-1, Icd-2, lgg,* and *Pgm*). This transect of fifteen quadrats was constructed in a shallow (5 m) region of the lake to enhance the accuracy of dredge placement. The length of the transect was chosen to approximate the length of the average site sampled in the original study (Table 7.2). The results from this fine-scaled sampling are given in Table 7.3. Wright's F_{IT} and F_{IS} statistics indicated a deficiency in heterozygotes within the transect and within quadrats. This clearly indicated small-scale population structure of the chironomid larvae.

Table 7.3. F_{IS}, F_{IT} and F_{ST} statistics for chironomid larvae collected from fifteen quadrats of a transect in Clear Lake (California). Modified from Table 4 of Woodward, Mulvey and Newman (1996)

Allozyme locus	F_{IS}	F-Statistic F_{IT}	F_{ST}
Aat	0.202	0.210	0.010
Ada	0.116	0.138	0.025
Est	0.024	0.247	0.019
gl	0.250	0.264	0.019
Hk	0.024	0.030	0.006
Icd-1	0.107	0.115	0.009
Icd-2	0.021	0.034	0.014
Igg	0.102	0.124	0.024
Pgm	0.010	0.020	0.011
Mean	0.134	0.150	0.018

Woodward, Mulvey and Newman (1996) concluded that a Wahlund effect, not mercury-related selection nor inbreeding, was the most likely explanation for the deficiencies of heterozygous genotypes. Their conclusion was based on the following observations and rules of logic:

(1) Departures from Hardy–Weinberg expectations involved a deficiency of heterozygotes (Hardy–Weinberg expectations and Selander's *D* values).

(2) There was no correlation between mercury contamination and genotype frequencies, i.e. no evidence of a cause–effect relationship nor a concentration–effect gradient.

(3) Ockham's razor (principle of parsimony) favors explanations with the fewest assumptions.

(4) Egg mass deposition patterns provide a mechanism for clustering of genetically distinct larvae as they settle nonrandomly onto the sediments.

(5) Wright's *F*-statistics suggest considerable structure along the mercury gradient and within the smaller-scale transect.

(6) There is no obvious obstacle to adult mating which would lead to inbreeding.

The potential for a Wahlund effect should always be kept in mind when interpreting population genetics data for populations exposed to toxicants.

Woodward Mulvey and Newman (1996) provide only one example of the importance of such thoughtfulness, but other examples exist. Lavie and Nevo (1986) suggested from laboratory testing that one could examine a suite of species and focus on the proportion of heterozygotes relative to homozygotes in populations. This conclusion was based on results from five gastropod species lethally exposed to cadmium and homozygote:heterozygote ratios for the enzyme, glucosephosphate isomerase, in survivors. They state that there seems to be a relationship for this proportion with pollution intensity and "[t]his pattern seems to have been established by natural selection". They attribute the difference in survival to the higher stability of the homodimer than the heterodimer of this dimeric enzyme: homozygotes had an enzyme form that was more resistant to inactivation by cadmium. Clearly, such an approach would be valid only in the demonstrated absence of a Wahlund effect.

Computer-intensive methods are now widely available to augment or to eventually replace the metrics just described for estimating gene flow and population structure. For example, a personal computer can now quickly produce bootstrap confidence intervals for F_{ST} (Rousset and Raymond 1997). Q-statistics (Nei 1973) can also be generated for structured populations in a manner analogous to performing statistical variance component analysis (Rousset and Raymond 1997; Bossart and Prowell 1998). More involved computer models incorporating geographical distances in algorithms allow more specific analysis of genetic data. For more information, the interested reader is directed to Bossart and Prowell (1998) who recently reviewed conventional and new means of assessing gene flow in structured populations.

7.3.5 MULTIPLE-LOCUS HETEROZYGOSITY AND INDIVIDUAL FITNESS

At this point, concepts related to neutral theory have been explored with the aim of demonstrating how toxicants can influence population genetics in the absence of differences in individual fitness. In the remainder of this chapter, two bridging topics will be mentioned between neutral theory and selection-based theory. The general consequences of different levels of heterozygosity of individuals will be discussed relative to overall fitness. Then long-term evolutionary consequences for species having decreased genetic diversity will be explored briefly.

Numerous studies have demonstrated that an individual's overall heterozygosity can influence its fitness. However, a number of publications have shown that it does not (e.g. Koehn, Diehl and Scott 1988). Multiple-locus heterozygosity refers here to the number of scored loci for which the individual is heterozygous. Relevant measures of fitness for which heterozygosity did influence fitness vary widely and include survival (Samallow and Soulé 1983; Pemberton et al. 1988), developmental rate (Danzmann et al. 1985, 1986 1988), developmental stability

(Ferguson 1986; Mulvey Keller and Meffe 1994), metabolic rate (Mitton, Carey and Kocher 1986, Danzmann Ferguson and Allendorf 1987) or metabolic cost (Garton, Koehn and Scott 1984), and growth rate (Koehn and Gaffney 1984; Garton, Koehn and Scott 1984; McAndrew, Ward and Beardmore 1986, Bush, Smouse and Ledig 1987). Mitton's recent book, *Selection in Natural Populations* (1997), provides extensive discussion of such correlations between fitness metrics and heterozygosity. Some studies suggest that heterozygosity can also influence susceptibility to toxicants, e.g. Nevo *et al.* (1986). However, careful analysis of one study of mercury toxicity (Diamond *et al.* 1989) and a similar study of arsenic toxicity (Newman *et al.* 1989) demonstrated that the observed relationships were artifacts reflecting the sum of individual locus effects, not an effect of heterozygosity *per se* (Newman *et al.* 1989). (Unfortunately, Table 6 of Gillespie and Guttman (1999) incorrectly lists the results of Diamond *et al.* (1989) and Newman *et al.* (1989) as supporting evidence for a relationship between heterozygosity and fitness.)

Why should there be a relationship between fitness and heterozygosity? There are three common explanations: inbreeding depression, multiple-locus heterosis, and optimal metabolic efficiency.

The inbreeding depression explanation can be understood from our discussions of inbreeding and heterozygosity. A decrease in heterozygosity can indicate increased inbreeding. Heterozygosity might simply be reflecting the degree of inbreeding experienced by individuals. Inbreeding can lead to lowered fitness (via inbreeding depression) as the probability of an individual being homozygous for deleterious genes increases. Low heterozygosity for the entire genome was approximated with scored loci and was correlated with a general inbreeding depression (Smouse 1986). Although plausible, Leary, Allendorf and Knudsen (1987) described one case in which inbreeding was not the explanation for the relationship between heterozygosity and a measure of individual fitness, developmental stability.

The multiple-heterosis explanation extends the phenomena of heterosis to include many loci. Single-locus heterosis is the superior performance of heterozygotes relative to homozygotes. It can also be defined in terms of hybrids (Zouros and Foltz 1987). The performance of hybrids produced from two lines is often superior to that of the two parent lines. Multiple-heterosis is the sum of heterotic effects at several loci. Heterozygosity will be positively correlated with hybrid vigor and can be envisioned as representing the opposite of the negative relationship just described between heterozygosity-correlated inbreeding and fitness.

Optimal metabolic efficiency may be linked to high fitness (Zouros and Foltz 1987; Dykhuizen, Dean and Hartl 1987). Individuals heterozygous for major glycolytic and Krebs cycle-related loci (enzymes typically used in these studies) may be more metabolically efficient or flexible than homozygous genotypes. Allozymes, allelic variants of enzymes, can differ in their properties, including kinetic properties (Hines *et al.* 1983) and resistance to toxicant inactivation (Kramer and Newman 1994). A homozygote at a particular locus will have only one form of the enzyme available but the heterozygote will have two (or more for multimeric enzymes) forms available. A homozygote, e.g. 100/100, for a dimeric enzyme will produce only one protein subunit and only one dimer will be produced. Heterozygotes, e.g. 100/165, synthesize two proteins (100 and 165) and three functional dimeric enzymes will be produced, 100/100, 100/165, and 165/165. Individuals with more heterozygous loci may have more metabolic options available to cope with changing environmental demands. Relative to their homozygous counterparts, highly heterozygous individuals might be more efficient over a wider range of conditions. If some allozymes are inactivated more readily than others by metals (Eichhorn 1974; Lavie and Nevo 1982; Kramer and Newman 1994) or are less tolerant to high temperatures (Zimmerman and Richmond 1981), an individual's fitness may be enhanced by having several forms present to catalyze essential reactions. Parsons (1997) provides a general review of stress and genetic variation.

**Box 7.4   Tolerance of fish to stressors increases with heterozygosity...
Sometimes**

Studies of allozyme variation by Guttman and co-workers (Kopp, Guttman and Wissing 1992; Schluetter *et al*. 1995) assessed the relationship between effects of stressor exposure and individual heterozygosity. Two of their studies will be used to demonstrate the variation possible in results from such studies.

Heterozygosity does influence sensitivity

Responses to high metal and low pH conditions were studied in populations of the central mudminnow (*Umbra limi*) (Kopp, Guttman and Wissing 1992). The concern addressed by this study was the consequence of acid precipitation on populations of fish endemic to the Adirondack Mountains (New York, USA). These researchers noted that individuals from waterbodies with high aluminum and low pH had higher levels of heterozygosity at enzyme-determining loci than those from reference sites. Slightly more than two hundred mudminnows from impacted and reference sites were exposed in the laboratory to assess whether mudminnows from contrasting sites responded similarly during acute exposure (96 h) to high aluminum (7.5 mg/L) and low pH (4.5) conditions. Pooling data for both sexes, Kopp, Guttman and Wissing (1992) found that the distribution of fish among three sensitivity classes (sensitive, intermediate, tolerant) was positively correlated with heterozygosity. These data supported the concept that measures of fitness tend to increase as individual heterozygosity increases.

Heterozygosity Does Not Influence Sensitivity

A statistically more robust experimental design was applied by Schluetter *et al*. (1995) to address the relationship between genetic variation at enzyme-determining loci and differential survival of more than a thousand fathead minnow (*Pimephales promelas*) exposed to copper. Survival time analyses were applied so the gross assignment of fish to sensitive, intermediate, and tolerant classes could be avoided. A model predicting survival time based on fish weight and number of heterozygous loci was produced and null hypotheses of insignificant effect of these two covariates tested with a χ^2 test. Although fish size was significantly ($\alpha = 0.05$) and positively related to survivorship, there was no apparent effect of number of heterozygous loci on survival of fathead minnows during copper exposure. These data clearly did not support the premise that measures of fitness tend to increase as individual heterozygosity increases. In another case, this failure to observe an effect could have been attributed to a lack of statistical power; however, the experiment involved large numbers of individuals and a powerful analysis technique.

7.4 GENETIC DIVERSITY AND EVOLUTIONARY POTENTIAL

Although discussed to this point as an indicator of population state or change, genetic diversity itself is crucial to the long-term viability of species populations. Mutation rates are extremely low relative to the rates of toxicant-accelerated drift, and the balance between drift and mutation is complex as evidenced by our above discussions. Regardless, an emerging concern of many population ecotoxicologists (e.g. Mulvey and Diamond 1991; Kopp, Guttman and Wissing 1992) is the ratcheting downward of genetic diversity due to neutral theory-related consequences of pollution. Because genetic variation is the raw material upon which natural selection works, the evolutionary potential of species might be lowered by toxicant exposure. Such long-term impacts of toxicant exposure are very difficult to quantify and are rarely addressed in the development of regulations.

7.5 SUMMARY

Several kinds of mechanism for DNA damage are described in this chapter, suggesting ample opportunity for direct mutagenic effects of toxicants on species germ lines. Indirect effects on the germ line are discussed based on neutral population genetic theory. In the absence of natural selection, modified stochastic processes as a consequence of toxicant exposure can have a profound impact on population genetic characteristics. The dynamics of such changes and tools for identifying them are described. Based on neutral theory, the potential for loss of genetic diversity is discussed. Ecotoxicology will benefit from incorporation of these concepts into the assessment of toxicant effects on populations. Natural selection as described in the next chapter could greatly modify these predictions of toxicant-driven reductions in genetic diversity (Mulvey and Diamond 1991).

7.5.1 SUMMARY OF FOUNDATION CONCEPTS AND PARADIGMS

- Toxicants which are mutagens can influence the germ line directly.
- Stochastic processes can influence the germ line.
- Hardy–Weinberg equilibrium in a population of diploid species is based on the assumptions of an effectively infinite population, no natural selection, and negligible mutation rates and migration rates. Violations of any of these assumptions can result in deviations from Hardy–Weinberg expectations.
- Genetic drift can be accelerated by a toxicant-related decrease in the effective population size. The decrease in effective population can result from toxicant effects on total population size, sex ratio, natality, mean generation time, population structure, and brood size variance.
- In addition to accelerated drift, abrupt decreases in effective population size can lead to abrupt genetic bottlenecks and consequent founder effects.
- Genetic diversity is maintained by a balance between mutation rate and drift. In a structured population, migration also influences genetic diversity.
- Effective population size is influenced by the distribution of individuals within a population.
- Sampling a cryptically structured population or the presence of migration into a population can result in an apparent deficit of heterozygotes, i.e. the Wahlund effect.
- Wright's F-statistics can be used to describe population genetic structure.
- Increases in multiple-locus heterozygosity are often, but not always, correlated with increases in individual fitness, including that associated with toxicant stress.
- Loss of genetic diversity due to toxicant exposure can reduce the evolutionary potential of a species population.

REFERENCES

Ayala FJ (1982). *Population and Evolutionary Genetics*. Benjamin/Cummings, Menlo Park, CA.

Baker RJ, Van den Bussche RA, Wright AJ, Wiggins LE, Hamilton MJ, Reat EP, Smith MH, Lomakin MD and Chesser RK (1996). High levels of genetic change in rodents of Chernobyl. *Nature* **380**: 707–708.

Baker RJ, Van den Bussche RA, Wright AJ, Wiggins LE, Hamilton MJ, Reat EP, Smith MH, Lomakin MD and Chesser RK (1997). High levels of genetic change in rodents of Chernobyl. *Nature* **390**: 100.

Beerli P (1998). MIGRATE. *http://evolution.genetics.washington.edu/lamarc/migrate.html*

Berrli P and Felsenstein J (1999). Maximum-likelihood estimation of migration rates and effective population numbers in two populations using a coalescent approach. *Genetics* **152**: 763–773.

Bootma D and Hoeijmakers JHJ (1994). The molecular basis of nucleotide excision repair syndromes. *Mutation Res* **307**: 15–23.

Bossart JL and Prowell DP (1998). Genetic estimates of population structure and gene flow: limitations, lessons and new directions. *TREE* **13**: 202–206.

Burdon RH (1999). *Genes and the Environment*. Taylor & Francis, Philadelphia, PA.

Bush RM, Smouse PE and Ledig FT (1987). The fitness consequences of multiple-locus heterozygosity: the relationship between heterozygosity and growth rate in pitch pine (*Pinus rigida Mill.*) *Evolution* **41**: 787–798.

Cavalli-Sforza LL and Bodmer WF (1971). *The Genetics of Human Populations*. WH Freeman and Company, San Francisco, CA.

Crow JF and Kimura M (1970). *An Introduction to Population Genetics Theory*. Harper & Row, New York.

Danzmann RG, Ferguson MM and Allendorf FW (1985). Does enzyme heterozygosity influence developmental rate in rainbow trout? *Heredity* **56**: 417–425.

Danzmann RG, Ferguson MM and Allendorf FW (1987). Heterozygosity and oxygen-consumption rate as predictors of growth and developmental rate in rainbow trout. *Physiol Zool* **60**: 211–220.

Danzmann RG, Ferguson MM and Allendorf FW (1988). Heterozygosity and components of fitness in a strain of rainbow trout. *Biol J Linn Soc* **33**: 219–235.

Danzmann RG, Ferguson MM, Allendorf FW and Knudsen KL (1986). Heterozygosity and developmental rate in a strain of rainbow trout (*Salmo gairdneri*). *Evolution* **40**: 86–93.

Diamond SA, Newman MC, Mulvey M, Dixon PM and Martinson D (1989). Allozyme genotype and time to death of mosquitofish, *Gambusia affinis* (Baird and Girard), during acute exposure to inorganic mercury. *Environ Toxicol Chem* **8**: 613–622.

De Finetti B (1926). Considerazioni matematiche sul l'ereditarieta mendeliana. *Metron* **6**: 1–41.

Dykhuizen DE, Dean AM and Hartl DL (1987). Metabolic flux and fitness. *Genetics* **115**: 25–31.

Eichhorn GL (1974). Active sites of biological macromolecules and their interaction with heavy metals. In *Ecological Toxicology Research. Effects of Heavy Metals and Organohalogen Compounds*, ed. by AD McIntyre and CF Mills, pp. 123–214. Plenum Press, New York.

Facemire CF, Gross TS and Guillette Jr LJ (1995). Reproductive impairment in the Florida panther: nature or nurture? *Environ Health Perspec* **103** (Suppl. 4): 79–86.

Ferguson MM (1986). Developmental stability of rainbow trout hybrids: genomic coadaptation or heterozygosity? *Evolution* **40**: 323–330.

Forbes VE (1999). *Genetics and Ecotoxicology*. Taylor & Francis, Inc., Philadelphia, PA.

Fraústo da Silva JJR and Williams RJP (1993). *The Biological Chemistry of the Elements. The Inorganic Chemistry of Life*. Clarendon Press, Oxford.

Garton DW, Koehn RK and Scott TM (1984). Multiple-locus heterozygosity and the physiological energetics of growth in the coot clam, *Mulinia lateralis*, from a natural population. *Genetics* **108**: 445–455.

Gillespie RB and Gutmann SI (1999). Chemical-induced changes in the genetic structure of populations: effects on allozymes. In *Genetics and Ecotoxicology*, ed. by VE Forbes, pp. 55–77. Taylor & Francis, Inc., Philadelphia, PA.

Hartl DL and Clark AG (1989). *Principles of Population Genetics*. Sinauer Associates Inc., Sunderland, MA.

Hillis DM, Mortiz G and Mable BK (1996). *Molecular Systematics*. Sinauer Associates, Inc., Sunderland, MA.

Hines BA, Philipp DP, Childers WF and Whitt GS (1983). Thermal kinetic differences between allelic isozymes of malate dehydrogenase (Mdh-B locus) of largemouth bass, *Micropterus salmoides*. *Biochem Genetics* **21**: 1143–1151.

Hoffman GR (1996). Genetic toxicology. In *Casarett and Doull's Toxicology. The Basic Science of Poisons*, ed. by CD Klaassen, 5h edn, pp. 269–300. McGraw-Hill Health Professions Division, New York.

Hoffmann AA and Parsons PA (1997). *Extreme Environmental Change and Evolution*. Cambridge University Press, Cambridge.

Jablonka, E, and Lamb M (1995). *Epigenetic Inheritance and Evolution*. Oxford: University Press, Oxford.

Koehn RK and Gaffney PM (1984). Genetic heterozygosity and growth rate in *Mytilus edulis*. *Mar Biol* **82**: 1–7.

Koehn RK, Diehl WJ and Scott TM (1988). The differential contribution by individual enzymes of glycolysis and protein catabolism to the relationship between heterozygosity and growth rate in the coot clam, *Mulinia lateralis*. *Genetics* **118**: 121–130.

Kopp RL, Guttman SI and Wissing TE (1992). Genetic indicators of environmental stress in central mudminnow (*Umbra limi*) populations exposed to acid deposition in the Adirondack Mountains. *Environ Toxicol Chem* **11**: 665–676.

Kramer VJ and Newman MC (1994). Inhibition of glucosephosphate isomerase allozymes of the mosquitofish, *Gambusia holbrooki*, by mercury. *Environ Toxicol Chem* **13**: 9–14.

Lamb T, Bickham JW, Gibbons JW, Smolen MJ and McDowell S (1991). Genetic damage in a population of slider turtles (*Trachemys scripta*) inhabiting a radioactive reservoir. *Arch Environ Contam Toxicol* **20**: 138–142.

Lavie B and Nevo E (1982). Heavy metal selection of phosphoglucose isomerase allozymes in marine gastropods. *Mar Biol* **71**: 17–22.

Lavie B and Nevo E (1986). Genetic selection of homozygote allozyme genotpyes in marine gastropods exposed to cadmium pollution. *The Sci Total Environ* **57**: 91–98.

Leary RB, Allendorf FW and Knudsen KL (1987). Differences in inbreeding coefficients do not explain the association between heterozygosity at allozyme loci and developmental stability in rainbow trout. *Evolution* **41**: 1413–1415.

McAndrew BJ, Ward RD and Beardmore JA (1986). Growth rate and heterozygosity in the plaice, *Pleuronectes platessa*. *Heredity* **57**: 171–180.

Mitton JB (1997). *Selection in Natural Populations*. Oxford University Press, Oxford.

Mitton JB, Carey C and Kocher TD (1986). The relation of enzyme heterozygosity to standard and active oxygen consumption and body size of tiger salamanders, *Ambysoma tigrinum*. *Physiol Zool* **59**: 574–582.

Mulvey M and Diamond SA (1991). Genetic factors and tolerance acquisition in populations exposed to metals and metalloids. In: *Metal Ecotoxicology. Concepts and Applications*, ed. by MC Newman, and AW McIntosh, pp. 301–321. Lewis Press, Chelsea, MI.

Mulvey M, Keller GP and Meffe GK (1994). Single- and multiple-locus genotypes and life-history responses of *Gambusia holbrooki* reared at two temperatures. *Evolution* **48**: 1810–1819.

Murdoch MH and Hebert PDN (1994). Mitochondrial DNA diversity of brown bullhead from contaminated and relatively pristine sites in the Great Lakes. *Environ Toxicol Chem* **8**: 1281–1289.

NCRP (National Council on Radiation Protection and measurements). (1993). *Risk Estimates for Radiation Protection*. NCRP Report 115. NCRP, Bethesda, MD.

Nei M (1973). Analysis of gene diversity in subdivided populations. *Proc Natl Acad Sci* **70**: 3321–3323.

Nevo E, Noy R, Lavie B, Beiles A and Muchtar S (1986). Genetic diversity and resistance to marine pollution. *Biol J Linn Soc* **29**: 139–144.

Newman MC (1995). *Quantitative Methods in Aquatic Ecotoxicology*. CRC/Lewis Publishers, Boca Raton, FL.

Newman MC (1998). *Fundamentals of Ecotoxicology*. CRC/Ann Arbor Press, Boca Raton, FL.

Newman MC, Diamond SA, Mulvey M and Dixon P (1989). Allozyme genotype and time to death of mosquitofish, *Gambusia affinis* (Baird and Girard) during acute toxicant exposure: a comparison of arsenate and inorganic mercury. *Aquat Toxicol* **15**: 141–156.

O'Brien SJ, Roelke ME, Marker L, Newman A, Winkler CE, Meltzer D, Colly L, Evermann JF, Bush M and Wildt DE (1987). Genetic basis for species vulnerability in the cheetah. *Science* **227**: 1428–1434.

Ouborg NJ, Piquot Y and van Groenendael JM (1999). Population genetics, molecular markers and the study of dispersal in plants. *J Ecol* **87**: 551–568.

Parsons PA (1997). Stress-resistance genotypes, metabolic efficiency and interpreting evolutionary change. In *Environmental Stress, Adaptation and Evolution*, ed. by R Bijlsma and V Loeschcke, pp. 291–305. Birkhäuser Verlag, Basel.

Pemberton JM, Albon SD, Guinness FE, Clutton-Brock TH and Berry RJ (1988). Genetic variation and juvenile survival in red deer. *Evolution* **42**: 921–934.

Rannala B and Hartigan J (1996). Estimating gene flow in island populations. *Genet Res* **67**: 147–158.

Rannala B and Mountain J (1997). Detecting immigration by using multilocus genotypes. *Proc Nat Acad Sci USA* **94**: 9197–9201.

Richardson BJ, Baverstock PR and Adams M (1986). *Allozyme Electrophoresis: A Handbook for Animal Systematics and Population Studies*. Academic Press, Sydney.

Robison SH, Cantoni O and Costa M (1984). Analysis of metal-induced DNA lesions and DNA-repair replication in mammalian cells. *Mutat Res* **131**: 173–181.

Rousset F and Raymond M (1997). Statistical analyses of population genetic data: new tools, old concepts. *TREE* **12**: 313–317.

Samollow PB and Soulé ME (1983). A case of stress related heterozygote superiority in nature. *Evolution* **37**: 646–649.

Schlueter MA, Guttman SI, Oris JT and Bailer AJ (1995). Survival of copper-exposed juvenile fathead minnows (*Pimephales promelas*) differs among allozyme genotypes. *Environ Toxicol Chem* **14**: 1727–1734.

Selander RK (1970). Behavior and genetic variation in natural populations. *Am Zool* **10**: 53–66.

Smouse PE (1986). The fitness consequences of multiple-locus heterozygosity under the multiplicative overdominance and inbreeding models. *Evolution* **40**: 946–957.

Spiess EB (1977). *Genes in Populations*. John Wiley, New York.

Stone R (1992). Can a father's exposure lead to illness in his children? *Science* **258**: 31.

Strittholt JR, Guttmann SI and Wissing TE (1988). Low levels of genetic variability of yellow perch (*Perca flavescens*) in Lake Erie and selected impoundments. In *The Biogeography of the Island Region of Western Lake Erie*, ed. by JF Downhower, pp. 246–257. Ohio State University Press, Columbus, OH.

Swofford DL and Selander RB (1981). BIOSYS-1: A FOTRAN program for the comprehensive analysis of electrophoretic data in population genetics and systematics. *J Hered* **72**: 281–283.

Theodorakis CW and Shugart LR (1999). Natural selection in contaminated environments: a case study using RAPD genotypes. In *Genetics and Ecotoxicology*, ed. by VE Forbes, pp. 123–149. Taylor & Francis, Inc., Philadelphia, PA.

Williams JG, Kubelik AR, Livak KJ, Rafalski JA and Tingey SV (1990). DNA polymorphisms amplified by arbitrary primers are useful as genetic markers. *Nucl Acids Res* **18**: 6531–6535.

Wilson EO and Bossert WH (1971). *A Primer of Population Biology.* Sinauer Associates, Inc., Sunderland, MA.

Woodward LA, Mulvey M and Newman MC (1996). Mercury contamination and population-level responses in chironomids: can allozyme polymorphism indicate exposure?*Environ Toxicol Chem* **15**: 1309–1316.

Wright S (1943). Isolation by distance. *Genetics* **28**: 114–138.

Wright S (1951). The genetical structure of populations. *Ann Eugen* **15**: 323–354.

Zasukhina GD, Vasilyeva IM, Sdirkova NI, Krasovsky GN, Vasyukovich LYa, Kenesariev UI and Butenko PG (1983). Mutagenic effect of thallium and mercury salts on rodent cells with different repair activities. *Mutat Res* **124**: 163–173.

Zimmerman, E,G. and Richmond MC (1981). Increased heterozygosity at the *Mdh*-B locus in fish inhabiting a rapidly fluctuating thermal environment. *Am Fish Soc* **110**: 410–416.

Zouros E and Foltz DW (1987). The use of allelic isozyme variation for the study of heterosis. In *Isozymes: Current Topics in Biological and Medical Research 13*, ed. by MC Rattazzi, JG Scandalios and GS Whitt, pp. 1–59. Alan R. Liss, Inc., New York.

8 Population Genetics: Natural Selection

8.1 OVERVIEW OF NATURAL SELECTION

Natural Selection acts exclusively by the preservation and accumulation of variations, which are beneficial under the organic and inorganic conditions to which each creature is exposed at all periods of life. (Darwin 1872)

8.1.1 GENERAL

Natural selection will now be described in order to complete our discussion of pollutant-influenced evolution. More specifically, natural selection resulting in microevolution will be explored. Microevolution is evolution within a species in contrast to macroevolution, which focuses on evolutionary processes and trends encompassing many species. Emphasis will be placed on microevolution leading to enhanced resistance.

The terms resistance and tolerance will be used interchangeably as done elsewhere (Weis and Weis 1989, Forbes and Forbes 1994, Newman 1998). Some authors object to this synonymy, reserving resistance to mean the enhanced ability to cope with toxicants due to genetic adaptation and tolerance to mean the enhanced ability to cope with toxicants due to physiological, biochemical, or some other acclimation.

Natural selection is the change in relative genotype frequencies through generations resulting from differential fitnesses of the associated phenotypes. Pertinent differences in phenotype fitness can involve viability (survival) or reproductive aspects of an individual's life. Natural selection has the same basic qualities regardless of the life cycle component(s) in which it manifests. It is a process with three required conditions and two consequences (Figure 8.1) as summarized by Endler (1986). The first requisite condition is the existence of variation among individuals relative to some trait. The second is fitness differences associated with differences in that trait, i.e. differences in survival or reproductive success among phenotypes. The third condition is inheritance: the trait must be heritable. Of course, another implied requisite is Thomas Malthus's that individuals in populations are capable of producing offspring in numbers exceeding those needed to simply replace themselves. Excess production of individuals in each generation combined with heritable differences in fitness among individuals have predictable consequences.

IF a population in a particular environment possesses

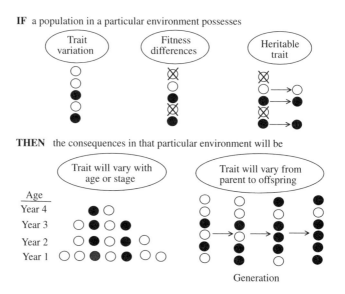

Fig. 8.1. Syllogism of natural selection (Endler 1986). If the three conditions of trait variation, trait-related fitness differences, and trait heritability exist, then the trait frequency will vary in a predictable manner among age/stage classes and generations of a population

As the first consequence of these three conditions, the frequency of a heritable trait will differ among age or life stage classes of a population. As detailed in Chapter 5, differences in survival and reproduction among individuals in demographic classes result in differences in the reproductive value (V_A) of individuals. This leads to the second consequence. The frequency of the trait from adult to offspring, i.e. across generations, will change due to trait-related differences in fitness. This change will be larger than expected due to random drift alone, i.e. due to stochastic processes alone. The net result is natural selection.

Differences in fitness can manifest in two ways. Differences may be controlled by one locus with the appearance of distinct fitness classes. In such cases of 'Mendelian genetics', one genotype may be intolerant, another tolerant and a third intermediate between the two. For example, Yarbrough *et al.* (1986) studied cyclodiene pesticide resistance in a population of mosquitofish (*Gambusia affinis*) endemic to an agricultural region of Mississippi and found resistance to be determined by a single, autosomal gene. Three distinct phenotypes were present for resistance. During acute cyclodiene exposure, resistance of heterozygotes (R/S) was intermediate to that of the sensitive (S/S) or resistant (R/R) homozygotes. Alternately, phenotype can be determined by several or many genes, resulting in a continuum of fitness states in a population. Such instances of 'quantitative traits' are treated differently from instances of Mendelian genetics, and the rate of adaptation is different than expected for a trait controlled by a single gene, e.g. selection is more rapid for traits under monogenic control versus those under polygenic control (Mulvey and Diamond 1991). Quantitative genetics methods for measuring toxicant-induced effects will be applied in Section 8.2.2 below.

Selection can be described as directional, stabilizing, or disruptive (Figure 8.2). Directional selection involves the tendency toward higher fitness at one side of the distribution of phenotypes (quantitative trait) or for a particular homozygous phenotype (Mendelian trait). The cyclodiene insecticide resistance in mosquitofish reported by Yarbrough *et al.* (1986) would result in directional selection. Stabilizing selection tends to favor intermediate phenotypes. Disruptive selection would favor the extreme phenotypes. Changes in the frequency of allozymes in pollution stressed gastropod species mentioned in Chapter 7 (Lavie and Nevo 1986a) suggested higher fitnesses of homozygotes than heterozygotes. In such a case, disruptive selection might be anticipated.

Several concepts associated with this overview of natural selection require comment at this point:

(1) Differences in fitness are specific to a particular environment and the relative fitnesses of genotypes can change if the environment changes sufficiently. Natural selection and fitness are specific to the environmental conditions under which individuals in the population exist, e.g. a species population that

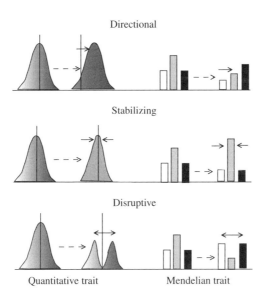

Fig. 8.2. An illustration of directional, stabilizing, and disruptive selection for quantitative (left side) and Mendelian (right side) traits. (Modified from Figure 1.3 of Endler (1986) and Figure 2 of Mulvey and Diamond (1991).)

has adapted successfully to an environmental toxicant will not necessarily be optimally adapted for a clean habitat.

(2) Natural selection leading to successful adaptation relative to one environment or environmental condition does not necessarily result in optimal adaptation for another environment or environmental condition. For example, adaptation to cope with a particular pollutant may not necessarily result in a population of individuals well adapted to another or to a natural stressor.

(3) Consistent, environment-specific differences in fitness are needed for natural selection to occur. Natural selection would not be possible if relative fitnesses of genotypes shifted randomly in direction and magnitude among generations. Natural selection can involve consistent relative fitnesses of genotypes or average relative fitness differences among genotypes in a fluctuating environment. The magnitude of the fitness differences may change somewhat, but the relative fitness of one genotype to another cannot abruptly and randomly change from one generation to another.

(4) Without sufficient genetic variability, a species population may fail to adapt and will become locally extinct.

(5) Because most environments are temporally and spatially variable, microevolution by natural selection can involve a population genome that shifts from one 'best obtainable' state to another.

Natural selection for traits or trait complexes within genetic subpopulations (demes) can impart to individuals within demes temporally and spatially defined optimal fitness, i.e. Wright's shifting balance theory (Wright 1932, 1982) (Figure 8.3). A species population occupying a landscape through time might be composed of many demes shifting continually to obtain the highest fitness of associated individuals. Demes continually climb toward the highest obtainable fitness peak in a changing 'adaptive landscape'. Random genetic drift allows the deme to explore the adaptive landscape and natural selection then moves the deme to the nearest optimal fitness peak. This process is repeated, resulting in demes that continually explore the adaptive landscape and establish themselves on obtainable adaptive peaks. According to Wright's shifting balance theory, there may be interdemic selection within a shifting landscape of environmental factors (Hoffmann and Parsons 1997). However, caution should be used when applying this last concept of interdemic selection, i.e. group selection working on competing demes within an adaptive landscape (Hartl and Clark 1989; Coyne, Barton and Turelli 1997, 2000). Although some studies suggest a certain amount of support (e.g. Ingvarsson 2000 and references therein), Sewall Wright's theory of interdemic selection is not been generally supported by observational nor experimental data. Regardless, important and relevant components of the shifting balance theory are demonstrably accurate (Coyne, Barton and Turelli 1997, 2000). The theory is mentioned here only to indicate that *through genetic drift and natural selection on individuals*, demes tend to shift continually within

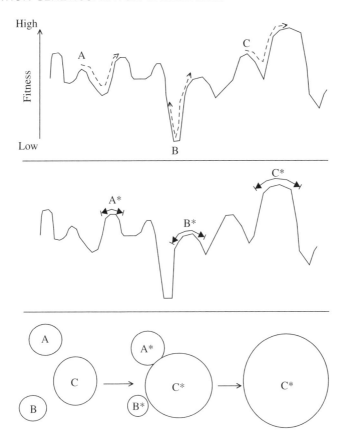

Fig. 8.3. Shifting balance theory (Wright 1932). The three phases of this theory combine genetic drift and natural selection to produce interdeme selection, i.e. group selection. Demes undergo genetic drift (top panel) which allows them to move from one adaptive peak through an adaptive valley to another peak (Phase I). Then, selection within demes maintains each at an adaptive peak (middle panel, Phase II). The best adapted deme will increase in size (number of individuals) and displace less well adapted demes (bottom panel, Phase III), i.e. selection of a group (deme). Although Phase III is not been supported by observational or experimental studies, Phase I and II are and can be important processes in natural populations (Coyne, Barton and Turelli 1997)

an adaptive landscape to occupy local peaks of optimal fitness. These peaks shift through time as the environment changes and natural selection *working on individuals* move the deme toward a new optimal fitness peak. Genetic drift allows exploration of nearby regions from a currently occupied fitness peak. Local populations under continual environmental pressure survive or even grow larger due to the increase in frequency of the most fit genotypes. It follows that demes will fail to adjust to changing environmental conditions unless they possess a certain level of genetic variation.

8.1.2 VIABILITY SELECTION

Perhaps the most conspicuous, and most commonly studied, type of selection by toxicants is that associated with differential survival, i.e. somatic viability of individuals. Viability selection can occur throughout the lifetime of an individual and includes fitness differences relative to development of the zygote, growth after birth, and survival to a sexual adult. For example, winter survival of juvenile red deer (*Cervus elaphus*) was correlated with allozyme genotype at several enzyme loci. Selection was implied from the observed fitness differences (Pemberton *et al.* 1988). A well-studied example involving pollution is the industrial melanism described in Chapter 2.

Differential survival is the most habitually studied quality in studies of pollutant-related viability. Many early studies involved the acquisition of tolerance to poisons in target and some nontarget species populations. Much of this work demonstrated rapid change of pest populations to chemicals applied to control them. Carson's *Silent Spring* (1962) includes many pages that discuss the rapid increase in survival of individuals in insect populations due to natural selection. Webb and Horsfall (1967) described the rapid decrease in pine mouse (*Pitymys pinetorum*) mortality after several years of control with endrin. Whitten, Dearn and McKenzie (1980) studied survival of insecticide-adapted sheep blowflies and Partridge (1979) described rodenticide (Warfarin) resistance in rats. Given this initial focus on the lose of pesticide efficacy, it is not surprising that survival came to dominate studies of adaptation to toxicants.

Much recent work with differential survival applied allozyme methods to identify tolerant or sensitive genotypes. Beardmore, Battaglia and co-workers (Battaglia *et al.* 1980; Beardmore 1980; Beardmore *et al.* 1980) and Nevo, Lavie and co-workers (Nevo *et al.* 1981; Lavie and Nevo 1982, 1986a,b) were among the first to apply these methods for exploring the genetic consequences of toxicant exposure for natural populations. In typical studies, field surveys were done to correlate allozyme genotype frequencies with degree of toxicant contamination. To augment these observations, individuals differing in allozyme genotypes were subjected to acutely toxic concentrations of toxicants in laboratory tests. The distribution of genotypes among survivors and dead individuals after exposure was used to imply differential fitness for the putative genotypes. The results would then be used to speculate about potential consequences to field populations exposed to much lower concentrations for longer periods of time. Speculation was normally based on the assumption that viability selection was the sole or most important component of selection and that differences noted at high concentrations reflect differences at low concentrations.

These allozyme-based experiments continue because allozyme genotypes are relatively easy to acquire and provide genetic markers for population processes. In

North America, Chagnon and Guttman (1989) and Gillespie and Guttman (1989) used this approach and suggested differential survival of mosquitofish (*Gambusia holbrooki*) and central stonerollers (*Campostoma anomalum*) of specific allozyme genotypes during acute exposure to metals. Results were compared to or used to imply a mechanism for changes in field populations. Similar studies also indicated differential fitness among acutely exposed, allozyme genotypes (e.g. Keklak, Newman and Mulvey 1994; Schlueter *et al.* 1995, 2000; Moraga and Tanguy 2000); however, the more powerful survival analysis methods introduced by Newman *et al.* (1989) and Diamond *et al.* (1989) were applied (see Chapter 3). Newman (1995) and Newman and Dixon (1996) provide details for analyzing such allozyme-survival time data. Mulvey and Diamond (1991) and Gillespie and Guttman (1999) provide reviews of studies relating allozyme genotype and toxicant exposure.

Box 8.1   Mercury, mosquitofish, metabolic allozyme genotype, and survival

Chagnon and Guttman (1989) suggested a relationship between survival of acute metal exposure and allozyme genotype but many crucial facets of this relationship remained unexplored. Studies of mosquitofish and mercury were undertaken to provide an in-depth study of allozyme genotype-related fitness effects during metal exposure and to examine the major qualities of such a relationship. In the first study (Diamond *et al.* 1989), nearly a thousand mosquitofish (*G. holbrooki*) were exposed to 0 mg/L or 1 mg/L inorganic mercury, and times-to-death were noted at 3- to 4-hour intervals for 10 days. The sex and wet weight of each fish were noted at death and individual fish were frozen for later allozyme analysis. In contrast to the negligible mortality in the reference tanks, 548 of 711 (77%) fish died in the mercury exposure tanks. Survival time methods were used to fit data to multivariate models (ln of time-to-death = f(fish wet weight, sex, genotypes at 8 isozyme loci)) and to test for significant effect ($\alpha = 0.05$) of the covariates on time-to-death. Not surprisingly, fish sex and size had significant influences on time-to-death: survival time was shorter for males than females and shortened as fish weight decreased. But a remarkable three of the eight isozyme loci (isocitrate dehydrogenase-1, *Icd-1*, malate dehydrogenase-1, *Mdh-1*, and glucosephosphate isomerase-2, *Gpi-2* = *Pgi-2*) had statistically significant effects on time-to-death. The first two of these enzymes are Krebs cycle enzymes and the last is a glycolytic enzyme.

A common explanation for relationships between allozymes and survival is that different genetically determined forms of the enzymes, e.g. different allozymes of GPI-2, differ in their capacity to bind metals and, consequently, to have their catalytic activities affected by metals. However, other studies (e.g. Watt, Carter and Blower 1985) suggest that, due to the crucial roles of these enzymes in metabolism, it was equally plausible that the different allozymes produced differences in metabolic efficiencies for stressed mosquitofish. Some genotypes might be metabolically more fit under stress than others. To assess these competing hypotheses, the experiment was repeated with a different toxicant (arsenate) which had a distinct mode of action, i.e. interference with oxidative phosphorylation. The binding of the oxyanion, arsenate, to enzymes would be quite different from that of the mercury cation. If binding with consequent enzyme dysfunction were the mechanism for the differential effect of mercury on *Gpi-2* genotypes, the trend noted for mercury-exposed fish would not be predicted for arsenate-exposed fish.

Also, it was possible that sampling of the fish from the source population unintentionally resulted in subsampling a structured population with lineages differing in tolerance and having more or less of one particular genotype by chance alone. Allozyme genotypes could merely be correlated with lineages that differed in their tolerances for one or more reasons (see Section 8.2.2 below). Mosquitofish reproductive and ecological characteristics combined with the highly structured pond from which the fish were taken reinforced this possibility. Another exposure study was done several months after the first during another annual reproductive pulse, allowing the source population time to grow and change structuring via lineages.

The results (Newman *et al.* 1989) indicated that the *Gpi-2* effect on time-to-death was present for arsenate as well as mercury exposure. The most sensitive genotype ($Gpi^{38/38}$) was the same for both toxicants. This suggested that the enzyme inactivation hypothesis was incorrect for the GPI-2 effect on survival. The relationships involving the other two loci were not seen again, suggesting that sampling artifacts from a structured source population likely produced these last two relationships. (See Lee, Newman and Mulvey 1992 below (Box 8.4) for supporting justification for this conclusion.)

Heagler *et al.* (1993) found this *Gpi-2* effect on time-to-death during mercury exposure to be consistent through time. Similar results were obtained when the mercury exposure was repeated several years after the Diamond *et al.* (1989) and Newman *et al.* (1989) studies. Their work further supported the premise that the *Gpi-2* effect was not an artifact associated with ephemeral population structuring. During the 1993 testing, groups of fish from the same source population were exposed to several mercury concentrations. Although GPI-2 did influence time-to-death at most concentrations, differences in allozyme fitness were obscured above a certain mercury concentration.

Kramer and Newman (1994) further tested the assumption that differential fitness of allozyme genotypes resulted from metal inactivation of the enzymes. Mosquitofish GPI-2 allozymes were partially purified and subjected *in vitro* to a series of mercury concentrations. The degree of inactivation of these *Gpi-2* allozymes was not correlated with the differential survival of the *Gpi-2* genotypes, suggesting again that inactivation was not the mechanism for the observed differential survival. Kramer *et al.* (1992a,b) also examined glycolysis and Krebs cycle metabolites in fish with different *Gpi-2* genotypes and found that the sensitive genotype (*Gpi-2*$^{38/38}$) displayed shifts in metabolism during exposure to mercury that were distinct from the other *Gpi-2* genotypes. These differences in allozyme genotype sensitivity were a function of metabolic differences under toxicant stress, not differences in metal binding to and inactivation of allozymes.

The results suggested that *Gpi-2* genotype frequencies might be useful as a marker of population-level response to stressors. However, potential effects of population structure, toxicant concentration, and intensity of other stressors must be understood and controlled in any such exercise. Also, as will be discussed in the next section, the potential for selection also occurring for reproductive traits could complicate prediction based solely on differences in survival.

8.1.3 SELECTION COMPONENTS ASSOCIATED WITH REPRODUCTION

Selection can occur at other equally important components of an organism's life cycle (Figure 8.4). This was evident from the very first elucidation of the concept of natural selection as evidenced by Charles Darwin's phrase 'at all periods of life' in the opening quote of this chapter. The first selection component (viability selection, SC1) involves survival differences and other fitness differences from zygote formation to sexual maturity. Viability selection could be measured for different age classes, e.g. Christiansen *et al.* (1974). There might be differences in development from zygote to a mature adult. These differences might involve survival or growth rates as discussed briefly in Chapter 6. Obviously, any increase in the probability of an individual reaching sexual maturity and surviving for a long period as a sexually active adult will also enhance reproductive success.

Selection component SC2 (sexual selection) in Figure 8.4 involves differential success of adults in finding, attracting, or retaining mates. For cxample, Watt, Carter and Blower (1985) found differential mating success in *Colias* butterflies that differed in genotype at a phosphoglucose isomerase (*Gpi*) locus. Like Kramer *et al.* (1992a,b) above, they attributed these differences in fitness to metabolic differences among *Gpi* genotypes. Sexual selection can occur for males (male sexual selection) or females (female sexual selection). Sexual selection might also involve differential success of mating pairs. Some genotype pairs may have a higher probability than others of being successful mates.

Three additional selection components involve the processes of gamete production and successful zygote formation. Meiotic drive (SC3) involves the differential production of the possible gamete types by heterozygotes. Sperm or ova may be

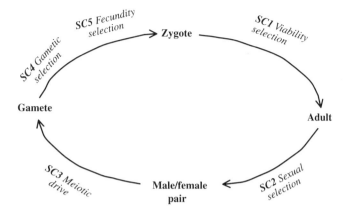

Fig. 8.4. Selection components in the life cycle of individuals. (See text for details)

produced with unequal allele representation by heterozygous individuals, leading to a higher probability of production of certain offspring genotypes. Gametic selection (SC4) can occur if certain gametes produced by heterozygotes have a higher probability of being involved in fertilization than others. Fecundity selection (SC5) can occur if pairs of certain genotypes have more offspring than others.

Endler (1986) makes the important observation that several selection components often co-occur and it is essential to understand the balance between fitnesses at these different components. A careful reexamination of Box 2.1 will show that a preoccupation at one point (adult predation by visual predators) distracted researchers for some time from selection at other life cycle stages (pre-adult survival). Prediction from one component (e.g. viability during acute toxicant exposure) can lead to inaccurate conclusions regarding selection consequences. In fact, there are indications that selection for reproductive components may be much more common than viability selection (Clegg, Kahler and Allard 1978; Nadeau and Baccus 1981).

Selection components analysis is possible for many species (e.g. Bungaard and Christiansen 1972; Christiansen and Frydenberg 1973; Christiansen, Frydenberg and Simonsen, 1973; Nadeau, Dietz and Tamarin 1981; Siegismund and Christiansen 1985; Williams, Anderson and Arnold 1990). The analysis requires known parent–offspring combinations and scoring of genotypes for a series of demographic classes, e.g. mother–offspring pairs, adult females (gravid or nongravid), and adult males. The sequence of hypotheses (Table IV of Christiansen and Frydenberg (Table 8.1)) are tested for these data with χ^2 statistics. The hypotheses in selection component analysis are tested sequentially and testing stops after a hypothesis is rejected. Each hypothesis test in the sequence is based

Table 8.1. Sequential hypotheses tested in selection component analysis. (From Table IV of Christiansen and Frydenberg 1973 as modified by Newman 1995)

Sequence	Hypothesis
First	Half of the offspring of heterozygous females are heterozygous. (implying that there is no selection among females gametes.) Rejection implies gametic selection.
Second	The frequency of transmitted males gametes is independent of the genotype of a female. Rejection of this hypothesis implies nonrandom mating with female sexual selection.
Third	The frequency of transmitted male gametes is equal to the frequency in adult males. Rejection implies differential male mating success and gametic selection in males.
Fourth	The genotype frequencies are equal among gravid and nongravid, adult females. Rejection implies differential female mating success.
Fifth	Genotype frequencies are equal for male and female adults. Rejection implies that zygotic (viability) selection is not the same for males and females.
Sixth	The adult genotype frequency is the same as that estimated for the zygotic population. Rejection implies zygotic (viability) selection.

on the assumption that the previously tested hypotheses were not 'false', i.e. not rejected in a statistical test.

Box 8.2   Selection components for mercury-exposed mosquitofish

Most studies of natural selection contain three major faults: (1) no estimates of life-time fitness; (2) consideration of only a few traits; and (3) unknown or poorly known trait function. (Endler 1986)

Our studies of mercury-exposed mosquitofish attempt to avoid the shortcomings described above by Endler. The glycolytic differences noted in mercury-exposed mosquitofish genotypes define a *Gpi-2* trait function potentially resulting in fitness differences. Points 1 and 2 will now be addressed.

The work of Mulvey *et al.* (1995) (Box 6.1) was used to illustrate the concepts of reaction norms and energy allocation trade-offs. Unsatisfied with predictions from the viability differences described in Box 8.1, Mulvey *et al.* (1995) used selection component analysis to explore the possibility of reproduction-related fitness differences in populations chronically exposed to mercury. This was possible because the mosquitofish is a prolific, live-bearing species amenable to mesocosm study and selection components analysis. Two mesocosm populations were grown with weekly additions of 18 µg/L of inorganic mercury and two mesocosm populations were grown in untreated water. After 111 days, all fish were collected and their sex, size, reproductive status (gravid/nongravid), and number of late stage embryos per gravid female determined. Selection components analysis as just described was performed for several allozyme loci; however, only *Gpi-2* results are relevant here. The methods of Christiansen, Frydenberg and Simonsen (1973) as implemented with the FORTRAN program listed in Appendix 29 of Newman (1995) were used to test a series of hypotheses like those in Table 8.2. As described in Box 6.1, rare *Gpi-2* alleles were combined in the analyses. An ANCOVA was then applied to the number of late-stage embryos carried by each gravid female to assess whether fecundity selection was occurring.

Table 8.2. Results of selection component analysis for the *Gpi-2* locus of mercury-exposed mosquitofish. (Modified from Table 4 in Mulvey *et al.* 1995.)

| Hypothesis | P-values from χ^2 test for each replicate mesocosm | | | |
	Control mesocosms		Mercury-spiked mesocosms	
Female gametic selection?	0.54	0.64	0.07	0.71
Random mating?	0.76	0.96	0.51	0.91
Male reproductive selection?	0.70	0.88	0.07	0.73
Female sexual selection?	0.55	0.52	**0.01**	**0.09**
Zygotic selection equal in sexes?	0.54	0.18	0.009	0.26
Zygotic selection?	0.68	0.19	0.42	0.58

Female sexual selection was suggested from the results of the selection component analysis (Table 8.2). For the two control mesocosms, P-values from the hypothesis testing (SC2) were 0.55 and 0.52. This suggested no female sexual selection was occurring under control conditions. However, the P-values for the mercury-spiked mesocosms were 0.01 and 0.09. These low P-values were taken to indicate female sexual selection and no further hypotheses were evaluated.

Whether a mature female was gravid or not was dependent on its *Gpi-2* genotype. Approximately 68–71% of females of all genotypes in all treatments, with one important exception, were gravid. Only 43% of *Gpi-2*$^{100/100}$ homozygous females were gravid in the mercury-spiked mesocosms. ANCOVA also indicated ($P = 0.01$) that, if gravid, a *Gpi-2*$^{100/100}$ female carried fewer developing embryos than the other genotypes.

These results indicating a reproductive disadvantage for *Gpi-2*$^{100/100}$ genotypes are particularly important because the genotype least likely to survive acute mercury exposure was the *Gpi-2*$^{38/38}$ homozygote. The potential exists for balancing selection components, i.e. viability selection balanced against female sexual and fecundity selection. Under some conditions, one component might outweigh another in determining the selection-driven changes in allele frequencies of a population. The results allowed a complete description of fitness differentials for several selection components, avoiding the second shortcoming listed above by Endler for studies of natural selection.

Aware that balancing selection was possible and that wild populations of mosquitofish experience wide variation in effective population size and migration, Newman and Jagoe (1998) conducted simulations of *Gpi-2* allele frequency changes in mosquitofish populations exposed acutely and chronically to mercury for many generations. In this way, overall fitness consequences (Endler's fault 1 above) could be defined more fully under different conditions. Results indicated that *Gpi-2* allele frequencies did change in predictable ways despite the potentially confounding effects of balancing selection, accelerated genetic drift, and migration. In general, viability selection seemed to overshadow reproductive selection components and toxicity-related acceleration of genetic drift. These results supported field studies by Heagler *et al.* (1993) suggesting that cautious use of *Gpi-2* as a marker of population-level effects was possible.

8.2 ESTIMATING DIFFERENTIAL FITNESS AND NATURAL SELECTION

To understand natural selection, and for predictive purposes, it is not sufficient merely to demonstrate that selection occurs; we need to know its rate, at least in the populations under study. Rates are estimated and predicted for selection coefficients and differentials. (Endler 1986)

8.2.1 FITNESS, RELATIVE FITNESS, AND SELECTION COEFFICIENTS

How are differences in fitness quantified? The conventional presentation of methods (Ayala 1982; Gillespie 1998) begins with a trait determined by one locus with two alleles, i.e. A_1 and A_2. Under the assumptions of the Hardy–Weinberg relationship, the A_1A_1, A_1A_2 and A_2A_2 genotype frequencies are predicted by $1 = q^2 + 2pq + p^2$ where $q =$ the A_1 allele frequency and $p =$ the A_2 allele frequency. However, equation (8.1) depicts the expected genotype frequencies if there are relative fitnesses to be considered for the three genotypes, w_{11}, w_{12}, w_{22}. Assume, for example, that fitness differences in viability are determined using the frequencies of A_1A_1, A_1A_2 and A_2A_2 genotype for neonates and then again for adults. The relationship among the genotypes for the neonates would be $1 = q^2 + 2pq + p^2$. However, prediction of genotype frequencies for adults would involve an additional factor — differential fitnesses:

$$\overline{w} = p^2 w_{11} + 2pq w_{12} + q^2 w_{22} \qquad (8.1)$$

where $\overline{w}$ = the average fitness for all genotypes. Equation (8.1) can be rearranged to normalize fitness to the average fitness:

$$1 = p^2 \frac{w_{11}}{\overline{w}} + 2pq \frac{w_{12}}{\overline{w}} + q^2 \frac{w_{22}}{\overline{w}} \tag{8.2}$$

Now, the frequencies of the three genotypes are predicted as a function of Hardy–Weinberg expectations (e.g. p^2) adjusted for the normalized fitness values (e.g. $w_{11}/\overline{w}$) of each genotype.

Predicted frequencies of alleles A_1 and A_2 after such selection are defined by equations (8.3) and (8.4) (Ayala 1982; Gillespie 1998):

$$p_1 = p^2 \frac{w_{11}}{\overline{w}} + pq \frac{w_{12}}{\overline{w}} \tag{8.3}$$

$$q_1 = pq \frac{w_{12}}{\overline{w}} + q^2 \frac{w_{22}}{\overline{w}} \tag{8.4}$$

The change in $p(\Delta_p = p_1 - p)$ and $q(\Delta_q = q_1 - q)$ frequencies per generation are predicted from equations (8.5) and (8.6) (Spiess 1977; Ayala 1982; Gillespie 1998):

$$\Delta_p = \frac{pq[p(w_{11} - w_{12}) + q(w_{12} - w_{22})]}{\overline{w}} \tag{8.5}$$

$$\Delta_q = \frac{pq[p(w_{12} - w_{11}) + q(w_{22} - w_{12})]}{\overline{w}} \tag{8.6}$$

The change in the average fitness can be estimated iteratively over many generations to visualize the changes due to selection in the population. According to Fisher's (1930) theorem of natural selection, higher levels of variation in fitness in populations will result in higher rates of change in the average fitness. The more variation in fitness in the population, the quicker the mean population fitness will increase under selection. Conversely, low variation results in slow or minimal selection. (See Hartl and Clark 1989 for details and equations for applying the above approach to multiple allele genes.)

Relative fitnesses can also be estimated for genotypes. The quotient of w for each genotype can be used with the w in the denominator being that for the most fit genotype, e.g. w_{11}/w_{11}, w_{12}/w_{11}, and w_{22}/w_{11} where A_1A_1 is assumed to have the highest fitness. These relative fitness values can also be expressed in terms of a selection coefficient ($s = 1 - w$ where w is the relative fitness value):

Genotype	Fitness(w)	Relative fitness	Selection coefficient (s)
A_1A_1	w_{11}	$w_{11}/w_{11} = 1$	$1 - (w_{11}/w_{11}) = 0$
A_1A_2	w_{12}	w_{12}/w_{11}	$1 - (w_{12}/w_{11})$
A_2A_2	w_{22}	w_{22}/w_{11}	$1 - (w_{22}/w_{11})$

As an example, selection against a recessive gene with a $w_{22} = 0.5$ would produce the following values:

Genotype	Fitness(w)	Relative fitness	Selection coefficient (s)
A_1A_1	$w_{11} = 1$	$w_{11}/w_{11} = 1$	$1 - (w_{11}/w_{11}) = 1 - 1 = 0$
A_1A_2	$w_{12} = 1$	$w_{12}/w_{11} = 1$	$1 - (w_{12}/w_{11}) = 1 - 1 = 0$
A_2A_2	$w_{22} = 0.5$	$w_{22}/w_{11} = 0.5/1 = 0.5$	$1 - (w_{22}/w_{11}) = 1 - 0.5 = 0.5$

Gillespie (1998) expresses selection by including a heterozygous effect (h). The relative fitness values for A_1A_1, A_1A_2 and A_2A_2 become $w_{11}/w_{11} = 1$, $w_{12}/w_{11} = $ 1-hs and $w_{22}/w_{11} = $ 1-s. The h is 0 if A_1 is completely dominant, 1 if A_1 is completely recessive, or between 0 and 1 if A_1 is partially recessive. Relationships described in equations (8.5) and (8.6) can be defined in terms of selection coefficients (i.e. Spiess 1977; Endler 1986). For example, if A_2 is recessive, $h = 0$, and selection is occurring for A_2, equation (8.7) (Endler 1986) is relevant:

$$\Delta_p = \frac{spq^2}{1 - sq^2} \tag{8.7}$$

Box 8.3 Relative fitness of mosquitofish genotypes exposed to mercury

After completing the studies described in Boxes 8.1 and 8.2, Newman and Jagoe (1998) developed computer models to assess the potential use of *Gpi-2* allele frequency changes as markers of population level effects. They explored the shifts in allele frequencies under different exposure scenarios. Many of the scenarios involved differential survival during acute mercury exposure and, consequently, estimates of relative fitness for exposed fish were needed. The approach of Newman (1995) was used to convert survival time model results to relative fitness values. The original time-to-death data were fit to a proportional hazard model (see Section 3.1.3.1 of Chapter 3) that included effects of fish sex, wet weight and *Gpi-2* genotype. The following equation describes the resulting model in terms of median time-to-death:

$$\text{MTTD} = e^{4.134}e^{0.358*\text{Sex}}e^{3.157*\text{Weight}}e^{\beta*\text{Genotype}}e^{-0.188}$$

where sex is 1 for females and 0 for males, weight is expressed in grams of wet weight, and genotype $= 0$ for *Gpi-2*$^{38/38}$ and 1 for all other genotypes. The last term ($e^{-0.188}$) was estimated from the model's estimated scale factor (σ) of 0.514 and the parameter for the median of a Weibull distribution (-0.36651), i.e. $e^{(0.514*-0.36651)}$. This allowed prediction of the median TTD. (See references in Chapter 3 for more details.) The β values (Table 8.3) were estimated for each genotype and reflect the sensitivity of each genotype relative to an arbitrary reference genotype (*Gpi-2*$^{38/38}$).

Table 8.3. Estimation of relative fitness values for mosquitofish *Gpi-2* genotypes. (Modified from Example 18 in Newman 1995)

Genotype	β	Relative risk	Relative fitness (w)	Selection coefficient (s)
100/100	0.370	$e^{-0.3700/0.514} = 0.487$	$0.402/0.487 = 0.82$	$1 - 0.82 = 0.18$
100/66	0.468	$e^{-0.468/0.514} = 0.402$	$0.402/0.402 = 1.00$	$1 - 1 = 0.00$
100/38	0.362	$e^{-0.362/0.514} = 0.494$	$0.402/0.494 = 0.81$	$1 - 0.81 = 0.19$
66/66	0.389	$e^{-0.389/0.514} = 0.469$	$0.402/0.469 = 0.86$	$1 - 0.86 = 0.14$
66/38	0.339	$e^{-0.339/0.514} = 0.517$	$0.402/0.517 = 0.78$	$1 - 0.78 = 0.22$
38/38	0	$e^{-0/0.514} = 1.000$	$0.402/1.000 = 0.40$	$1 - 0.40 = 0.60$

The above model is a proportional hazard model: the hazard to each genotype was constant through time and the relative hazards of one genotype to any other remain constant. This allows the expression of the β coefficients as relative risks: relative risk = $e^{\beta/\sigma}$. These relative risks are estimates of genotype fitness which can be transformed to relative fitness values by simply dividing the relative risk of the most tolerant genotype by the relative risk of each genotype. The *Gpi-2*$^{66/100}$ was the most tolerant genotype as its relative risk was the smallest of all genotypes, so 0.402 is divided by all genotypes' relative risks to estimate relative fitness values (w) for each genotype. These differences in w and s values were quite large. Hartl and Clark (1989) indicate that selection coefficients with as small a difference as 1% can have very significant influence on allele frequencies in a population.

These calculations allowed the results of the toxicity trial to be included in conventional genetic models to predict changes in allele frequencies under selection. The further inclusion of reproductive differences in fitness during chronic exposures (i.e. Box 8.2) allowed predictions based on the combination of viability selection during acute exposure, and female sexual and fecundity selection during chronic exposure to mercury.

8.2.2 HERITABILITY

Heritability of polygenetic traits can be quantified under the assumption that variation in the phenotypes expressed among individuals results from a combination of genetic variation, environmental variation, and perhaps, the interaction or covariation of genetic and environmental factors (Figure 8.5):

$$\sigma_p^2 = \sigma_g^2 + \sigma_e^2 + \sigma_{g\times e}^2 \qquad (8.8)$$

where $\sigma_p^2 =$ the phenotypic variance, $\sigma_g^2 =$ the genetic variance, $\sigma_e^2 =$ the environment-related variance, and $\sigma_{g\times e}^2 =$ the variance due to the genetic $\times$ environment interaction. This last component is more accurately called the covariance between genetic and environmental factors. The environmental

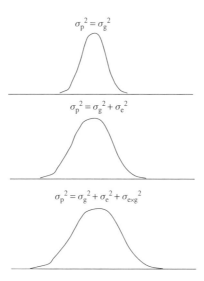

Fig. 8.5. The components contributing to the variance in a phenotypic trait. (See text for details)

component (σ_e^2) includes differences among phenotypes due to diverse environmental factors such as nutrition, microhabitat, and developmental conditions. The genetic component (σ_g^2) of the phenotypic variance can be separated into the additive variance arising from genetic factors (σ_a^2), a dominance component accounting for the influence of differences in gene dominances (σ_d^2), and epistatic variance (σ_i^2). The additive component is simply the sum of the effects of each of the individual genes contributing to the phenotype. The dominance component includes the influence of gene dominance on phenotypic expression. Potential epistatic interactions among relevant genes are included in σ_i^2:

$$\sigma_p^2 = \sigma_a^2 + \sigma_d^2 + \sigma_i^2 + \sigma_e^2 + \sigma_{g\times e}^2 \qquad (8.9)$$

Three simplifying assumptions are applied initially in many studies of heritability: (1) quantitative traits are often normally distributed (Ayala 1982; Gillespie 1998), (2) gene × environment covariance can be ignored initially, and (3) only additive effects need be considered (i.e. equation (8.10)). Notice that the first assumption of a normally distributed, quantitative trait is inconsistent with the individual effective dose or individual tolerance hypothesis described in Box 2.2 which assumes a lognormal distribution for toxicant tolerance. Notice also that, because the dominance component (σ_d^2) of the total phenotype variance is not subject to individual selection, it is not necessary to include it below (equation (8.11)) in estimating heritability:

$$\sigma_p^2 = \sigma_a^2 + \sigma_e^2 \qquad (8.10)$$

In such a case, the narrow sense heritiability (h^2) is simply the additive variance divided by the phenotypic variance:

$$h^2 = \frac{\sigma_a^2}{\sigma_p^2} \tag{8.11}$$

Narrow sense heritability can be estimated using linear regression of the measured trait of offspring (dependent variable) versus that of a parent who shares half of its genes (independent variable). For example, the quantitative trait of interest (e.g. time-to-death in an acute toxicity test) is measured for the mother and also for her offspring. This is done for many parent–offspring pairs and a regression slope (b) calculated using least squares regression. The regression slope (b) is used to estimate h^2 because $b = h^2/2$. Division by 2 is required here because only half of the genes in the offspring are shared with its mother.

Heritability can also be estimated using experiments designed around twins and sibs (Ayala 1982; Spiess 1977). Alternately, the mean of a trait for both parents ('midparent trait') can be compared to that of offspring (Spiess 1977). Although these methods are rarely applied in ecotoxicology, Klerks and Levinton (1989) estimated the heritability of metal tolerance for the oligochaete, *Limnodrilus hoffmeisteri*, using regression of the log of the midparent survival time versus the log of the mean offspring survival time. Heritability estimates indicated high levels of heritable variation for metal tolerance. McNeilly and Bradshaw (1968) provide a similar example of estimating heritability for plants species exposed to heavy metals. Posthuma *et al.* (1993) estimated heritability of metal tolerance for a soil springtail (*Orchesella cincta*) by employing a variety of these methods.

The qualifier 'narrow sense' is applied above to heritability without any explanation. This phrase is added to distinguish it from the more inclusive, broad sense heritability. Broad sense heritability (H^2) includes the other components defined in equation (8.9):

$$H^2 = \frac{\sigma_g^2}{\sigma_p^2} = \frac{\sigma_a^2 + \sigma_d^2 + \sigma_i^2}{\sigma_p^2} \tag{8.12}$$

Being the proportion of the total phenotypic variation attributable to all genetic components, broad sense heritability simply indicates the amount of genetic influence on the trait (Spiess 1977).

Box 8.4 Phenotype variance and heritability of mosquitofish exposed to mercury

> In studying allozyme effects on time-to-death of mosquitofish (*Gambusia holbrooki*) acutely exposed to mercury, Newman, Mulvey and co-workers became concerned about the amount of phenotypic variation (time-to-death) due to environmental, genetic, and genetic × environment interactions (see

Boxes 8.1 to 8.3 for details). The wild caught fish used for these experiments were collected from an abandoned farm pond with dense masses of submerged vegetation. As adult mosquitofish readily consume new-born mosquitofish, clutches of newly born mosquitofish tend to remain hidden in nearby vegetation until they are large enough not to be readily eaten. This clustering of broods in vegetation clumps could create discrete lineages that are captured in a biased manner with dip netting. If high frequencies of some allozyme genotypes are correlated with specific broods, spurious correlations may occur between allozyme genotypes and time-to-death. Perhaps environmental or genetic × environmental interactions produce lineages that differ in phenotype, not allozyme genotype. Earlier correlations between time-to-death and genotypes at two allozyme loci (Diamond *et al.* 1989; Newman *et al.* 1989) were found to be temporally inconsistent (Heagler *et al.* 1993). To address this possibility of spurious correlations due to temporally variable lineages, Lee, Newman and Mulvey (1992) did the following experiment with fish from the reference population. Central to the analysis of the results are the concepts of sources of phenotypic variation and heritability.

Gravid females were dip netted from the reference pond and placed into 40 L tanks. They were allowed to give birth to young that were transferred to 120 L plastic pools. Each pool contained one brood (sibship) and all pools were situated adjacent to one another outdoors. This isolation of broods in adjacent pools simulated the spatial isolation occurring in the reference pond.

The mothers were placed into separate, perforated containers suspended in an exposure tank three weeks after producing their broods. Each female's time-to-death was then recorded during exposure to 1 µg/L of mercury. These times-to-death were later compared to those of their offspring.

Offspring were reared as described above until they reached sexual maturity. Females from each brood were exposed as just described for their mothers and the average brood time-to-death calculated for each sibship. Males were omitted from exposures and later comparison to their mothers because previous studies (Diamond *et al.* 1989; Newman *et al.* 1989) showed that time-to-death differed between males and females.

Narrow sense heritability was estimated by linear regression of mother versus average daughter times-to-death, i.e. $b = h^2/2$. The slope of the resulting regression line was not significantly different from 0, i.e. no narrow sense heritability was detected.

The environmental effects associated with sibship isolation during development was also assessed by applying analysis of covariance (ANCOVA) to time-to-death data for daughters. Included in the model were sibship ('Brood') and mean wet weight of exposed daughters in each sibship. There was a highly significant effect of sibship ($P = 0.004$) on time-to-death of the daughters. (The F-test for significant effect of wet weight on time-to-death resulted in a $P = 0.070$.)

These analyses indicate that sharing of a mother and a common habitat during maturation influenced phenotype (time-to-death), but there was no evidence of an additive genetic component to this variation. The concerns of Lee *et al.* (1992) regarding the potential influence of lineage on correlations between time-to-death and allozyme genotypes were quite justified.

8.3 ECOTOXICOLOGY'S TRADITION OF TOLERANCE

. . .it was the advent of DDT and all its many relatives that ushered in the true Age of Resistance. (Carson 1962)

Populations exposed to toxicants and not eliminated outright may eventually display increased tolerance given sufficient fitness differences, selection pressure, and time. Tolerance may be gaged with one or more phenotypic traits such as enhanced survival, development, growth, or reproduction. However, enhanced tolerance will not emerge and the local population will become extinct in the absence of sufficient genetic variation relative to tolerance, consistent selection pressure for tolerance, and sufficient time.

Key factors influencing the process of tolerance acquisition are summarized in Table 8.4 (modified from Table 1 in Mulvey and Diamond (1991)). Genetic qualities influencing tolerance acquisition include initial allele frequencies, dominance, number of genes involved in determining the tolerance phenotype, and the magnitude of the fitness differences among genotypes. Tolerance acquisition will be slower if it involves a rare allele instead of a more common allele. Also, there is a higher risk of allele loss if the allele is initially rare in a population experiencing high levels of mortality as can be the case in toxicant-exposed populations. If the tolerance gene is dominant, tolerance will emerge rapidly relative to the case in which it is associated with a recessive gene. As an example, Yarbrough and colleagues (Chambers and Yarbrough 1979; Wise, Yarbrough and Roush 1986; Yarbrough *et al.* 1986) demonstrated enhanced pesticide tolerance of mosquitofish (*Gambusia affinis*) in agricultural areas. Pesticide resistance in mosquitofish was defined by one dominant gene. In another example, Martínez and Levinton (1996) found rapid metal tolerance acquisition controlled by a single gene in an oligochaete population.

Consistent with Fisher's theorem of natural selection (see Section 8.2.1), the rate of change in the average tolerance of the population increases as the genetic variability of the tolerance trait in the initial population increases (e.g. equations (8.5) and (8.6)). The larger the difference in fitness among the genotypes, the faster the increase in average population tolerance will occur. The industrial melanism of the peppered moth (Box 2.1) is a clear example of rapid microevolution due to the large fitness differences among color morphs and dominance of dark over light color morphs. As described in Sections 8.1.2 and 8.1.3, selection can occur at different stages of an organism's life cycle. Selection

Table 8.4. Factors influencing the rate at which tolerance is acquired in populations

Quality	Description of influence
Genetic qualities	
Allele frequency	Tolerance will increase more rapidly if the tolerance allele is common, not rare, in the population before selection begins.
Gene dominance	Tolerance increases more rapidly in early generations if the tolerance allele is dominant.
Monogenic or polygenic	Tolerance will increase more rapidly if controlled by one gene versus many genes.
Fitness differences	Tolerance will increase more rapidly if differences in fitness among genotypes are large (versus small).
Selection components	Selection at different components of a life cycle can negate directional selection for one tolerance trait by counterbalancing selection for another trait, or accelerate the rate of selection for tolerance traits by reinforcing the advantage of a particular genotype.
Co-tolerance	Preadaptation to a toxicant can result in elevated tolerance in a population if adaptation took place in the past for a related toxicant, e.g. a plant population adapted to one herbicide is later exposed to a similar herbicide.
Reproductive qualities	
Generation time	Tolerance will increase more rapidly for species with short generation times versus long generation species.
Intrinsic rate of increase	Tolerance will increase more rapidly for populations with high intrinsic rates of increase versus populations with low intrinsic rates of increase.
Size of population (N_e)	Genetic variation decreases with a decrease in N_e. Consequently, large populations will have more variation in tolerance and the possibility of tolerance increasing is higher for large populations versus small populations.
Ecological qualities	
Migration	Influx of nontolerant genotypes due to immigration can slow the rate of tolerance acquisition: Increased levels of migration will slow tolerance acquisition.
Refugia	The presence of refugia, i.e. uncontaminated habitat, allows intolerant individuals to remain in the population and can slow the rate of tolerance acquisition.
Life stage sensitivity	Selection effectiveness can be influenced by the most sensitive life stage.

at one component of an organism's life cycle can counterbalance selection for a tolerance trait associated with another component of the organism's life cycle. Previous discussion of longevity (antagonistic pleiotropy in Chapter 6) illustrates the importance of life cycle stage on favoring or not favoring a particular trait. On the other hand, if tolerance traits at different selection components disfavor the same genotypes, tolerance acquisition can be accelerated due to the reinforcing of the genotype disadvantage by several tolerance traits. Therefore, it is critical to understand all selection components before making predictions about tolerance acquisition. Finally, a previous adaptation to one toxicant can result in cross-resistance or co-tolerance. This co-tolerance can result in very rapid accommodation to a novel toxicant. For example, plants tolerant to a particular s-triazine herbicide produce a herbicide-binding protein that can impart an elevated level of tolerance if these adapted plants are later exposed to a novel s-triazine herbicide (Erickson, Rahire and Rochaix 1985). Isopod tolerance to copper imparts a co-tolerance to lead (Brown 1978).

Factors other than genetics influence tolerance acquisition. Short generation time and rapid population growth rates increase the rate of tolerance acquisition. Effective population size and the associated changes in population genetic variability influence selection for tolerance. All else being equal, larger populations generally possess more genetic variability than smaller ones and, consequently, the chance of enhanced tolerance emerging and the rate of tolerance change will be higher for larger than for smaller populations. Relative to metapopulation considerations, an increase in migration into an exposed population will slow the rate at which the average population tolerance increases (e.g. Newman and Jagoe 1998). The presence of refugia or source demes of nontolerant genotypes will also slow the rate at which average tolerance level increases in the exposed population.

A rich literature describes toxicant-related tolerance in natural populations. Those focused on plants are particularly thorough, e.g. Antonovics (1971), Pitelka (1988), Wilson (1988), Baker and Walker (1989) and Macnair (1997). Good reviews exist for the topic relative to insect resistance to pesticides (e.g. Mallet 1989) and animal tolerance to pollutants (e.g. Klerks and Weis 1987; Klerks 1990; Mulvey and Diamond 1991; Forbes and Calow 1997).

8.4 SUMMARY

In this brief chapter the characteristics and dynamics of microevolution were described relative to natural selection and tolerance acquisition. The conditions giving rise to and the consequences of natural selection were defined. The genetic dynamics of demes are explored using parts of Wright's shifting balance theory, especially the complementary exploration of the adaptive landscape afforded by genetic drift and the shift onto adaptive peaks due to natural selection. Selection components were described and the importance of exploring all relevant selection components emphasized. Metrics of differential fitness and selection coefficients were explored as were those for narrow and broad sense heritability. Finally, tolerance acquisition was described relative to fundamental factors influencing rates of increase for average population tolerance.

8.4.1 SUMMARY OF FOUNDATION CONCEPTS AND PARADIGMS

- Genetic drift and natural selection are complementary processes giving rise to evolutionary change.

- Natural selection is the change in relative genotype frequencies through generations due to differential fitnesses of the associated phenotypes. Pertinent differences in phenotype fitness can involve viability or reproductive aspects of an individual's life.

- Four required conditions for natural selection are the following: (1) the existence of variation among individuals relative to some trait, (2) fitness differences associated with differences in that trait, (3) heritability of that trait, and (4) the Malthusian premise that individuals in populations can produce excess offspring.

- There are two consequences of the four conditions for natural selection. The frequency of a heritable trait will differ among age or life stage classes. Also, the frequency of the trait from adult to offspring, i.e. across generations, will differ due to trait-related differences in fitness.

- Fitness differences may be controlled by one locus with the appearance of distinct fitness classes (Mendelian trait) or by several or many genes, resulting in a continuum of fitness phenotypes in a population (quantitative trait).

- Natural selection can be directional, disruptive, or normalizing.

- Differences in fitness are specific to a particular environment and the relative fitness of genotypes can change if the environment changes.

- Consistent, environment-specific differences in fitness are needed for natural selection to occur.

- Lacking sufficient, appropriate genetic variability, a species population may fail to adapt and will become locally extinct.

- Wright argued that, through genetic drift and natural selection on individuals, demes tend to shift continually within an adaptive landscape to occupy local fitness peaks. These peaks shift through time as the environment changes and natural selection working on individuals move the deme toward a new optimal fitness peak.

- Selection can occur at several stages of an organism's life cycle. Selection components include viability selection, sexual (male and female) selection, meiotic drive, gametic selection, and fecundity selection.

- Viability selection includes fitness differences in development of the zygote, growth after birth, and survival.

- Four other selection components involve reproduction. Sexual selection involves differences in adult success in finding, attracting, or retaining a mate. Meiotic drive involves the differential production of the possible gamete types by heterozygotes. Gametic selection occurs if certain gametes produced by heterozygotes have a higher probability of being involved in fertilization than others. Fecundity selection occurs if pairs of certain genotypes have more young than others.

- Selection for several selection components often occurs, making it essential to understand the net balance between fitnesses at these different components. Prediction from one component (e.g. viability during acute toxicant exposure) can lead to inaccurate predictions of selection consequences.

- Differences in fitness can be quantified as fitness (w), relative fitness, or selection coefficients (s).

- Heritability can be quantified by assuming that phenotypic variation among individuals results from a combination of genetic variation (including additive-, epistatic- and dominance-associated variance), environmental variation and, perhaps, the interaction between genetic and environmental factors.

- Narrow sense heritiability (h^2) is the additive genetic variance divided by the total phenotypic variance and broad sense heritability (H^2) includes the other variance components as defined in equation (8.9).

- The rate of tolerance acquisition in an exposed population is a function of genetic, ecological, and reproductive factors as summarized in Table 8.4.

REFERENCES

Antonovics J (1971). Metal tolerance in plants. In Cragg, J.B. (ed.). *Advances in Ecological Research, Volume 7*, ed. by JB Cragg, pp. 1–85. Academic Press, New York.

Ayala FJ (1982). *Population and Evolutionary Genetics*. Benjamin/Cummings, Menlo Park, CA.

Baker AJM and Walker PL (1989). Physiological responses of plants to heavy metals and the quantification of tolerance and toxicity. *Chem Spec Bioavail* **1**: 7–18.

Battaglia JA, Bisol PM, Fossato VU and Rodino E (1980). Studies of the genetic effect of pollution in the sea. *Rapp P-v Reun, Cons Int Explor Mer* **179**: 267–274.

Beardmore JA (1980). Genetical considerations in monitoring effects of pollution. *Rapp P-v Reun, Cons Int Explor Mer* **179**: 258–266.

Beardmore JA, Barker CJ, Battaglia B, Payne JF and Rosenfeld A (1980). The use of genetical approaches to monitoring biological effects of pollution. *Rapp P-v Reun, Cons Int Explor Mer* **179**: 299–305.

Brown BE (1978). Lead detoxification by a copper-tolerant isopod. *Nature* **276**: 388–390.

Bungaard J and Christiansen FB (1972). Dynamics of polymorphism, I: selection components in an experimental population of *Drosophilia melanogaster*. *Genetics* **71**: 439–460.

Carson R (1962). *Silent Spring*. Houghton Mifflin, New York.

Chagnon NL and Guttman SI (1989). Differential survivorship of allozyme genotypes in mosquitofish populations exposed to copper or cadmium. *Environ Toxicol Chem* **8**: 319–326.

Chambers JE and Yarbrough JD (1979). A seasonal study of microsomal mixed-function oxidase components in insecticide-resistant and susceptible mosquitofish, *Gambusia affinis*. *Toxicol Appl Pharmacol* **48**: 497–507.

Christiansen FB and Frydenberg O (1973). Selection component analysis of natural polymorphisms using population samples including mother–offspring combinations. *Theor Popul Biol* **4**: 425–445.

Christiansen FB, Frydenberg O and Simonsen V (1973). Genetics of *Zoarces* populations: IV. Selection component analysis of an esterase polymorphism using population samples including mother–offspring combinations. *Hereditas* **73**: 291–304.

Christiansen FB, Frydenberg O, Gyldenholm AO and Simonsen V (1974). Genetics of *Zoarces* populations, VI: further evidence based on age group samples, of a heterozygote deficit in the EST III polymorphism. *Hereditas* **77**: 225–236.

Clegg MT, Kahler AL and Allard RW (1978). Estimation of life cycle components of selection in an experimental plant population. *Genetics* **89**: 765–792.

Coyne JA, Barton NH and Turelli M (1997). Perspective: A critique of Sewall Wright's shifting balance theory of evolution. *Evolution* **51**: 643–671.

Coyne JA, Barton NH and Turelli M (2000). Is Wright's shifting balance process important in evolution? *Evolution* **54**: 306–317.

Darwin C (1872). *The Origin of Species*. Penguin Putnam Inc., New York.

Diamond SA, Newman MC, Mulvey M, Dixon PM and Martinson D (1989). Allozyme genotype and time to death of mosquitofish, *Gambusia affinis* (Baird and Girard), during acute exposure to inorganic mercury. *Environ Toxicol Chem* **8**: 613–622.

Endler JA (1986). *Natural Selection in the Wild*. Princeton University Press, Princeton, NJ.

Erickson JM, Rahire M and Rochaix J-D (1985). Herbicide resistance and cross-resistance: changes at three distinct sites in the herbicide-binding protein. *Science* **228**: 204–207.

Fisher RA (1930). *The Genetical Theory of Natural Selection*. Clarendon Press, Oxford.

Forbes VE and Calow P (1997). Responses of aquatic organisms to pollutant stress: theoretical and practical implications. In *Environmental Stress, Adaptation and Evolution*, ed. by R Bijlsma and V Loesohke, pp. 25–41. Birkhäuser Verlag, Basel.

Forbes VE and Forbes TL (1994). *Ecotoxicology in Theory and Practice*. Chapman and Hall, London.

Gillespie JH (1998). *Population Genetics. A Concise Guide*. The Johns Hopkins University Press, Baltimore, MD.

Gillespie RB and Guttman SI (1989). Effects of contaminants on the frequencies of allozymes in populations of the central stoneroller. *Environ Toxicol Chem* **8**: 309–317.

Gillespie RB and Gutmann SI (1999). Chemical-induced changes in the genetic structure of populations: effects on allozymes. In *Genetics and Ecotoxicology*, ed. by VE Forbes, pp. 55–77. Taylor & Francis, Inc., Philadelphia, PA.

Hartl DL and Clark AG (1989). *Principles of Population Genetics*. Sinauer Associates Inc., Sunderland, MA.

Heagler MG, Newman MC, Mulvey M and Dixon PM (1993). Allozyme genotype in mosquitofish, *Gambusia holbrooki*, during mercury exposure: temporal stability, concentration effects and field verification. *Environ Toxicol Chem* **12**: 385–395.

Hoffmann ΛΛ and Parsons PA (1997). *Extreme Environmental Change and Evolution*. Cambridge University Press, Cambridge.

Ingvarsson PK (2000). Differential migration from high fitness demes in the shining fungus beetle, *Phalacrus substriatus*. *Evolution* **54**: 297–301.

Keklak MM, Newman MC and Mulvey M (1994). Enhanced uranium tolerance of an exposed population of the eastern mosquitofish (*Gambusia holbrooki*, Girard 1859). *Arch Environ Contam Toxicol* **27**: 20–24.

Klerks PL (1990). Adaptation to metals in animals. In *Heavy Metals Tolerance in Plants: Evolutionary Aspects*, ed by AJ shaw, pp. 311–321. CRC Press, Boca Raton, FL.

Klerks PL and Levinton JS (1989). Rapid evolution of metal resistance in a benthic oligochaete inhabiting a metal-polluted site. *Biol Bull* **176**: 135–141.

Klerks PL and Weis JS (1987). Genetic adaptation to heavy metals in aquatic organisms: a review. *Environ Pollut* **45**: 173–205.

Kramer VJ and Newman MC (1994). Inhibition of glucosephosphate isomerase allozymes of the mosquitofish, *Gambusia holbrooki*, by mercury. *Environ Toxicol Chem* **13**: 9–14.

Kramer VJ, Newman MC, Mulvey, M and Ultsch GR (1992a). Glycolysis and Krebs cycle metabolites in mosquitofish, *Gambusia holbrooki*, Girard 1859, exposed to mercuric chloride: allozyme genotype effects. *Environ Toxicol Chem* **11**: 357–364.

Kramer VJ, Newman MC and Ultsch GR (1992b). Changes in concentrations of glycolysis and Krebs cycle metabolites in mosquitofish, *Gambusia holbrooki*, induced by mercuric chloride and starvation. *Environ Biol Fish* **34**: 315–320.

Lavie B and Nevo E (1982). Heavy metal selection of phosphoglucose isomerase allozymes in marine gastropods. *Mar Biol* **71**: 17–22.

Lavie B and Nevo E (1986a). Genetic selection of homozygote allozyme genotypes in marine gastropods exposed to cadmium pollution. *The Sci Total Environ* **57**: 91–98.

Lavie B and Nevo E (1986b). The interactive effects of cadmium and mercury pollution on allozyme polymorphisms in the marine gastropod, *Cerithium scabridum*. *Mar Pollut Bull* **17**: 21–23.

Lee CJ, Newman MC and Mulvey M (1992). Time to death of mosquitofish *(Gambusia holbrooki)* during acute inorganic mercury exposure: population structure effects. *Arch Environ Contam Toxicol* **22**: 284–287.

Mallet J (1989). The evolution of insectide resistance: have the insects won? *TREE* **4**: 336–340.

Macnair MR (1997). The evolution of plants in metal-contaminated environments. In *Environmental Stress, Adaptation and Evolution*, ed. by R Bijlsma and V Loeschke, pp. 3–24. Basel, Switzerland: Birkhäuser Verlag.

Martínez DE. and Levinton J (1996). Adaptation to heavy metals in the aquatic oligochaete *Limnodrilus hoffmeisteri*: evidence for control by one gene. *Evolution* **50**: 1339–1343.

McNeilly T and Bradshaw AD (1968). Evolutionary processes in populations of copper-tolerant *Argostis tenuis* Sibth. *Evolution* **22**: 108–118.

Moraga D and Tanguy A (2000). Genetic indicators of herbicide stress in the Pacific oyster *Crassostrea gigas* under experimental conditions. *Environ Toxicol Chem* **19**: 706–711.

Mulvey M and Diamond SA (1991). Genetic factors and tolerance acquisition in populations exposed to metals and metalloids. In *Metal Ecotoxicology. Concepts & Applications*, ed. by MC Newman and AW McIntosh, pp. 301–321, Chelsea, MI: Lewis Publishers.

Mulvey M, Newman MC, Chazal A, Keklak MM, Heagler MG and Hales Jr LS (1995). Genetic and demographic responses of mosquitofish (*Gambusia holbrooki*, Girard 1859) populations stressed by mercury. *Environ Toxicol Chem* **14**: 1411–1418.

Nadeau JH and Baccus R (1981). Selection components of four allozymes in natural populations of *Peromyscus maniculatus*. *Evolution* **35**: 11–20.

Nadeau JH, Dietz K and Tamarin RH (1981). Gametic selection and the selection component analysis. *Genet Res* **37**: 275–284.

Nevo E, Perl T, Beiles A and Wool D (1981). Mercury selection of allozyme genotypes in shrimps. *Experientia* **37**: 1152–1154.

Newman MC (1995). *Quantitative Methods in Aquatic Ecotoxicology*. Lewis/CRC Press, Boca Raton, FL.

Newman MC (1998). *Fundamentals of Ecotoxicology*. Ann Arbor/Lewis/CRC Press, Boca Raton, FL.

Newman MC, Diamond SA, Mulvey M and Dixon P (1989). Allozyme genotype and time to death of mosquitofish, *Gambusia affinis* (Baird and Girard) during acute toxicant exposure: a comparison of arsenate and inorganic mercury. *Aquat Toxicol* **15**: 141–156.

Newman MC and Dixon PM (1996). Ecologically meaningful estimates of lethal effect in individuals. In *Ecotoxicology. A Hierarchical Treatment*, ed. by MC Newman and CH Jagoe, pp. 225–253. Lewis/CRC Press, Boca Raton, FL.

Newman MC and Jagoe RH (1998). Allozymes reflect the population-level effect of mercury: simulations of mosquitofish (*Gambusia holbrooki*, Girard) GPI-2 response. *Ecotoxicology* **7**: 141–150.

Partridge GG (1979). Relative fitness of genotypes in a population of *Rattus norvegicus* polymorphic for Warfarin resistance. *Heredity* **43**: 239–246.

Pemberton JM, Albon SD, Guinness FE, Clutton-Brock TH and Berry RJ (1988). Genetic variation and juvenile survival in red deer. *Evolution* **42**: 921–934.

Pitelka LF (1988). Evolutionary responses of plants to anthropogenic pollutants. *TREE* **3**: 233–236.

Posthuma L, Hogervorst RF, Joose NG and van Straalen NM (1993). Genetic variation and covariation for characteristics associated with cadmium tolerance in natural populations of the springtail *Orchesella cincta* (L.). *Evolution* **47**: 619–6)31.

Schlueter MA, Guttman SI, Duan Y, Oris JT, Huang X and Burton GA (2000). Effects of acute exposure to fluoranthene–contaminated sediment on the survival and genetic variability of fathead minnows (*Pimephales promelas). Environ Toxicol Chem* **19**: 1011–1018.

Schlueter MA, Guttman SI, Oris JT and Bailer AJ (1995). Survival of copper-exposed juvenile fathead minnows (*Pimephales promelas*) differs among allozyme genotypes. *Environ Toxicol Chem* **14**: 1727–1734.

Siegismund HR and Christiansen FB (1985). Selection component analysis of natural polymorphisms using population samples including mother–offspring combinations, III. *Theor Popul Biol* **27**: 268–297.

Spiess EB (1977). *Genes in Populations.* John Wiley, New York.

Walker CH, Hopkin SP, Sibly RM and Peakall DB (1996). *Principles of Ecotoxicology.* Taylor & Francis, London.

Watt WB, Carter PA and Blower SM (1985). Adaptation at specific loci. IV. Differential mating success among glycolytic allozyme genotypes of *Colias* butterflies. *Genetics* **109**: 157–175.

Webb RE and Horsfall Jr F (1967). Endrin resistance in the pine mouse. *Science* **156**: 1762.

Weis JS and Weis P (1989). Tolerance and stress in a polluted environment: the case of the mummichog. *BioScience* **39**: 89–95.

Whitten MJ, Dearn JM and McKenzie JA (1980). Field studies on insecticide resistance in the Australian sheep blowfly, *Lucilia cuprina. Aust J Biol Sci* **33**: 725–735.

Williams CJ, Anderson WW and Arnold J (1990). Generalized linear modeling methods for selection component experiments. *Theor Popul Biol* **37**: 389–423.

Wilson JB (1988). The cost of heavy-metal tolerance: an example. *Evolution* **42**: 408–413.

Wise D, Yarbrough JD and Roush TR (1986). Chromosomal analysis of insecticide resistant and susceptible mosquitofish. *J Hered* **77**: 345–348.

Wright S (1932). The roles of mutation, inbreeding, crossbreeding and selection in evolution. *Proc 6th Int Cong Genet* **1**: 356–366.

Wright S (1982). The shifting balance theory and macroevolution. *Ann Rev Genet* **16**: 1–19.

Yarbrough JD, Roush RT, Bonner JC and Wise DA (1986). Monogenic inheritance of cyclodiene resistance in mosquitofish, *Gambusia affinis. Experientia* **42**: 851–853.

9 Conclusion

To conceive of it with a total apprehension I must for the thousandth time approach it as something totally strange. (Thoreau 1859, cited in Bickman 1999)

9.1 GENERAL

This small volume has explored ecotoxicology from the vantage of the population. Detail relative to populations was provided to enhance the reader's differentiation and integration of population-related information (see Chapter 1). This volume also bridges concepts and techniques in the next two series volumes, *Organismal Ecotoxicology* and *Community Ecotoxicology*. Hopefully, by this initial effort to translate concepts and metrics among hierarchical levels, consilience might gradually emerge as a strategic goal of ecotoxicology during the next decades.

Let's consider for the moment what has been presented in this volume. The vantage of population ecotoxicology, the science of contaminants in the biosphere and their effects on populations, was argued to be crucial for predicting extinction risk for populations under contaminant exposure. Such prediction is a central objective of much environmental legislation. With the exception of federal acts focused on human health or endangered species, the intent of key US environmental laws is assurance of species population viability in environments containing toxicants. This can be done more directly with population-based concepts and data than with individual-based concepts, models, and information. Potential contributions to the potential effectiveness of prediction can be found in the subdisciplines of epidemiology, population dynamics, demography, metapopulation biology, life history theory, and population genetics. Related concepts and techniques afford effective description and prediction of population consequences.

9.2 SOME PARTICULARLY KEY CONCEPTS

9.2.1 EPIDEMIOLOGY

Epidemiology provided a mode of describing toxicant-related disease in populations and quantitatively comparing disease in different populations or study groups. Models identifying risk factors for individuals within population were described, including proportional hazard, accelerated failure, and binary logistic regression models. Methods were demonstrated with examples of human disease; however, they are easily applied to other species.

Results from epidemiological studies also contribute to predicting genetic consequences of exposure, i.e. population consequences, as described for mercury-exposed mosquitofish (Chapter 8). Epidemiological studies also allow convenient estimation of mortality rates applied in simple population growth models, demographic life tables, and metapopulation models of exposed populations.

Interpretation of epidemiological results is susceptible to logical errors so evaluation of results has to be done thoughtfully. The foundations of causality were quickly reviewed. The intent was to describe common errors so that they might be avoided and, to borrow a phrase, to cultivate a 'wisdom of insecurity' (Watts 1968) about cause–effect relationships. Hill's aspects of disease association were explored as a specific set of rules commonly used to improve the process of identifying disease associations. Hill's rules are not the only ones relevant to ecotoxicology. The reader may also want to review those of Fox (1991) and Evans (1976). Because of the difficulty in assigning causality, formal Bayesian methods of enhancing belief would be extremely valuable in epidemiological surveys by ecotoxicologists. General references for Bayesian methods include Howson and Urbach (1989), Box and Tiao (1992), Retherford and Choe (1993), and Josephson and Josephson (1996). These methods are useful at all levels of the ecological hierarchy.

The possibility of contaminants influencing the infectious disease process in populations was explored briefly. The paradigm that toxicants increase the risk of infectious disease by weakening hosts (Odum 1971, 1985) was judged to be less inclusive than the disease triad paradigm (Figure 3.5). Toxicants, as components of the environment in which the host and parasite/pathogen are interacting, can favor either the host or parasite/pathogen. Infectious disease may be fostered or discouraged by exposure to toxicants.

9.2.2 SIMPLE MODELS OF POPULATION DYNAMICS

Phenomenological models of population dynamics were explored in Chapter 4, assuming a homogeneous distribution of identical individuals. They provided important insights despite the aggregation of information into basic parameters. Models allowed a clearer understanding of contaminant influence on the temporal dynamics of populations than afforded by conventional, individual-based methods. Some population effects noted during ecological risk assessments would be inexplicable or only vaguely explicable without such an understanding. Density-independent mortality due to toxicant exposure was added to classic population growth models. The possibility of enhanced population productivity ('yield') as well as reduced productivity was demonstrated with the inclusion of toxicant exposure into models used to predict yield for harvested fish and wildlife populations. Methods for estimating population consequences and time to recovery were described based on these basic models.

9.2.3 METAPOPULATION DYNAMICS

The consequences of uneven distribution of individuals in a contaminated environment were explored with metapopulation models. The risk of local population extinction or lowered carrying capacity were assessed most accurately with this metapopulation context, a context only now being introduced into ecotoxicology (O'Connor 1996).

It is crucial to understand the source–sink dynamics of the habitat mosaic populated by a species. Some poor habitats can contain a number of individuals only if a source habitat is nearby and individuals move among habitats. Keystone habitats and corridors for migration among segments of the population become crucial to predicting population consequences of contaminant exposure. Accurate prediction also depends on knowledge of other important population qualities within a landscape mosaic such as potential propagule rain and rescue effects. The metapopulation context also provides explanation for toxicant effects to individuals outside of the contaminated area.

9.2.4 THE DEMOGRAPHIC APPROACH

Applying basic demographic techniques, discussion moved beyond phenomenological models to include heterogeneity among individuals. Lamentably, much of the lethality and reproductive information currently generated for regulatory purposes — for protecting populations in contaminated habitats — is not gathered in a manner directly useful in demographic methods. Despite the discouragingly slow evolution of standard methods relative to effectively generating and applying ecotoxicology data to prediction of population consequences, demographic methods are being used with increasing frequency in ecotoxicology. Techniques consistent with demographic methods exist for analyzing toxicological data, e.g. the survival time and LTRE (Caswell 1996) methods. Simple and matrix-based demographic methods were described and means of including stochastic aspects of population projections were discussed.

Although applied widely by ecotoxicologists today, the most sensitive stage paradigm was identified as a false paradigm (weakest link incongruity). Predictions relying on demographic metrics such as age- or stage-dependent reproductive value should replace those based on the most sensitive stage paradigm.

9.2.5 LIFE HISTORY THEORY

Although emergent properties may confound predictions, life history theory can link contaminant-related changes in phenotype to population vital rates (Kooijman, Vander Hoeven and Van der Werf 1989; Sibly and Calow 1989; Calow and Sibly 1990; Sibly 1996). The principle of allocation suggests that an individual with a specific genetic make-up and living in a particular environment must allocate energy resources so as to maximize Darwinian fitness. Therefore, predictable rules for energy allocation should be identifiable, albeit expressed slightly differently, for individuals within populations. Shifts in energy allocation under different environmental conditions produce differences in population vital rates. For example, a contaminant may require increased energy expenditure for detoxification and repair of soma in order for an individual to survive to reproductive age. Once arriving at sexual maturity, that individual might have less energy reserve available for reproduction. Adjustment in the rate at which an individual becomes reproductively viable might also occur. There could be other life history changes. Such effects taken together for all individuals in a population result in changes in vital rates that could result in a change in population vitality or risk of local extinction.

Reaction norms define environment-dependent shifts in phenotype, i.e. phenotypic plasticity. Reaction norms can be inflexible in which case phenotype does not change once it is expressed. Some reaction norms can change during the life of an individual. Reaction norms for life history characteristics allow exploration of toxicant-induced shifts affecting population vital rates (e.g. Box 6.2).

Polyphenism occurs if an environmental cue triggers expression of one phenotype or another with no intermediate phenotypes being expressed. Polyphenisms are directly relevant to assessing effects of endocrine-modifying contaminants on population consequences. As an example, exposure to an endocrine-modifying contaminant could determine the sex of hatchlings that will make up the next generation of a turtle population.

Developmental stability is a valuable population-level metric quantifying the ability of individuals in a population to develop into a narrow range of phenotypes within a particular environment. Beyond a certain level of variation, deviations in phenotype expression imply a decrease in fitness of associated individuals. Metrics such as fluctuating asymmetry allow easy detection of changes in developmental stability due to contaminant exposure.

9.2.6 POPULATION GENETICS – STOCHASTIC PROCESSES

Population genetics can be affected by toxicant exposure. Direct changes to DNA can occur and, unless repaired, these changes led to the appearance of mutations. Stochastic processes determining genetic qualities of populations can also be influenced by contaminants. Contaminants can modify the spatial distribution of individuals within the population, effective population size, mutation rate, and migration rate.

Several quantitative tools allow assessment of stochastic consequences to population genetics. The Hardy–Weinberg principle predicts genotype frequencies if (1) the population is a large one of randomly mating individuals, (2) no natural selection is occurring, (3) mutation rates are negligible, and (4) migration rates are negligible. Deviations from Hardy–Weinberg expectations indicate violation of one or more of these conditions. Models of genetic drift as a function of effective population size allow prediction of genetic change with toxicant-induced reduction in population size. Selander's D-statistics quantifies the deficiency of heterozygotes. Those deficiencies could be a function of selection, inbreeding, or population structure, e.g. a Wahlund effect. Wright's F-statistics can provide understanding of the genetic structure of a population potentially composed of many demes or having genetic clines. Insight about normal genetic structure is necessary for properly interpreting genetic trends seen in field populations. Finally, genetic diversity itself is crucial to the long-term viability of species populations. Without variation, a population lacks the raw material with which to adapt to changes in its environment and will eventually disappear when the environment changes.

9.2.7 POPULATION GENETICS – NATURAL SELECTION

Natural selection can be another important process occurring in populations exposed to contaminants. It can result in enhanced tolerance, the enhanced ability to cope with toxicants due to physiological, biochemical, anatomical, or some other genetically based change in phenotype. However, natural selection resulting in enhanced tolerance requires genetic variation in the tolerance trait and populations lacking adequate variability are at higher risk of extinction than those with adequate variability.

Viability selection is often the focus of tolerance studies; however, other important selection components can be involved. They include male and female sexual selection, meiotic drive in heterozygotes, gametic selection in heterozygotes, and fecundity selection. Several selection components can occur simultaneously, perhaps resulting in balancing one component against another. It is important in predicting consequences of toxicant-driven selection that all potential selection components be assessed carefully.

9.3 CONCLUDING REMARKS

Hopefully, this short treatment of population ecotoxicology has been simultaneously informative and convincing. Several of the key concepts or relationships described here broaden one's understanding of toxicant effects in ecological systems. Many were clarified for me only after years of haunting my research program with Dr Margaret Mulvey. Hopefully, this book will allow the reader to move ahead without as many worrisome, conceptual 'bumps in the night' as I experienced. Also I hope that the reader is convinced of the importance of the population context in scientific and practical ecotoxicology.

REFERENCES

Box GEP and Tiao GC (1992). *Bayesian Inference in Statistical Analysis*. John Wiley, New York.
Calow P and Sibly RM (1990). A physiological basis of population processes: ecotoxicological implications. *Funct Ecol* **4**: 283–288.

Caswell H (1996). Demography meets ecotoxicology: untangling the population level effects of toxic substances. In *Ecotoxicology. A Hierarchical Treatment*, ed. by MC Newman and CH Jagoe, pp. 255–292. CRC/Lewis Press, Boca Raton, FL.

Evans AS (1976). Causation and disease: the Henle–Koch postulates revisited. *Yale J Biol Med* **49**: 175–195.

Fox GA (1991). Practical causal inference for ecoepidemiologists. *J Toxicol Environ Health* **33**: 359–373.

Howson C and Urbach P (1989). *Scientific Reasoning. The Bayesian Approach*. Open Court, La Salle, IL.

Josephson JR and Josephson SG (1996). *Abductive Inference. Computation, Philosophy, Technology*. Cambridge University Press, Cambridge.

Kooijman SALM, Van der Hoeven N and Van der Werf DC (1989). Population consequences of a physiological model for individuals. *Funct Ecol* **3**: 325–336.

O'Connor RJ (1996). Toward the incorporation of spatiotemporal dynamics into ecotoxicology. In *Population Dynamics in Ecological Space and Time*, ed. by OE Rhodes Jr, RK Chesser and MH Smith. The University of Chicago Press, Chicago, IL.

Odum EP (1971). Fundamentals of Ecology. WB Saunders Co., Philadelphia, PA.

Odum, EP (1985). Trends expected in stressed ecosystems. Bioscience **35**: 419–422.

Retherford RD and Choe MK (1993). *Statistical Models for Causal Analysis*. John Wiley, New York.

Sibly RM (1996). Effects of pollutants on individual life histories and population growth rates. In *Ecotoxicology. A Hierarchical Treatment*, ed. by MC Newman and CH Jagoe, pp. 197–223. CRC/Lewis Press, Boca Raton, FL.

Sibly RM and Calow P (1989). A life-history theory of responses to stress. *Biol J Linn Soc* **37**: 101–116.

Thoreau HD (1859). Quote from Bickman M (ed.) (1999). *Henry Thoreau on Education*. Houghton Mifflin, Boston, MA.

Watts AW (1968). *The Wisdom of Insecurity*. Random House, New York.

Index

.